Your Pregnancy Day by Day

Dr. Stuart Campbell

and Alison Mackonochie

Ballantine Books
New York

A Ballantine Books Trade Paperback Original

Copyright © 2005 by Carroll & Brown Limited

Managing Art Editor Emily Cook
Designer Laura de Grasse

All rights reserved.

Published in the United States by Ballantine Books, an imprint of The Random House Publishing Group, a division of Random House, Inc., New York.

BALLANTINE and colophon are registered trademarks of Random House, Inc.

Originally published in Great Britain by Carroll & Brown Publishers Limited, London.

The Library of Congress Cataloging-in-Publication Data is available upon request.

ISBN 0-345-48510-6

Reproduced by Colourscan, Singapore
Printed and bound in Singapore by SNP

www.ballantinebooks.com

987654321

Introduction

The approximately 280 days of a "normal" pregnancy are among the most memorable in a woman's life. From the minute she finds out that she is expecting, a pregnant woman becomes eager to know everything that will ensure an enjoyable pregnancy, a safe delivery, and a healthy baby.

Not only will this book help you do all that – it will also make you aware of how your baby develops, what he can do, and how he looks while you're waiting for him to be born.

You will find on each page of the diary, practical information on all aspects of pregnancy, labor, and delivery – from what you should eat, how you should exercise, the lifestyle choices you should make, and what you can do to ease any complaints, through to choices in childbirth, the different methods of pain relief during labor, and what happens during delivery. And, for those mothers whose babies don't arrive on their estimated dates of delivery, there are two extra weeks of useful information. Though the book is not a definitive guide to pregnancy, it will give you lots of useful information in an easily digestible form.

During the early weeks of development, the progress of your growing baby is illustrated by artwork, which more clearly shows the minute changes taking place. Once these weeks have passed, alongside of the daily advice to the mother, you will find an ultrasound image of a baby of the appropriate age and an explanation of his stage of development or behavior. I'm sure you will be delighted by the great range of expressions and actions of which babies are capable. You can be sure that your baby is looking very similar to, and doing the same things as, the babies shown.

Of course, not all babies develop at exactly the same rate and there are differences in length and weight, but doctors are generally agreed about the normal course of development. Therefore, in each of the pregnancy weeks, you can expect your baby to have acquired the abilities and appearance as cataloged over the course of the days of that week and to be approximately the length and weight as expressed in the week's vital statistics.

There is a difference, however, between the duration of pregnancy and that of gestation. Because pregnancy is dated from your last menstrual period and conception usually happens two weeks later, doctors count the weeks of pregnancy 14 days in advance of your baby's actual gestation. Therefore, during the 27th week of pregnancy, for example, your baby will be 24 weeks' gestational age until the end of the week, when he attains his 25th week.

YOUR MENSTRUAL CYCLE

Your pregnancy is dated from the first
day of your last menstrual cycle. The cycle
starts on the first day of menstrual bleeding
and lasts for around 28 days. At about day five
of your cycle an egg (ovum) starts to mature
inside a fluid-filled sac (follicle) in one of
your two ovaries and the lining of the uterus
becomes thicker in preparation for the
implantation of the egg if it becomes fertilized.
At around day 14 ovulation takes place. This is
when the egg is released into the Fallopian tube ready
to be fertilized. The egg remains ready for fertilization for
between 12 and 24 hours. If it is left unfertilized it is shed, along with the
lining of the uterus (endometrium), during the next menstrual period and the
whole process begins again. If fertilization takes place, you will be four weeks
pregnant by the time your next menstrual cycle is due to start again.

Fimbriae

Ripe ovum

Fallopian tube

Ovary

Endometrium

Developing egg follicle

Uterine cavity

SPERM

For fertilization to take place a sperm has to penetrate and fuse with the nucleus of the egg. Sperm are manufactured in the testes at a rate of about 125 million each day. Each sperm is made up of three parts: a head which contains the nucleus where the 23 chromosomes are stored; an acrosome cap, which enables the sperm to penetrate the egg, and a tail which allows it to swim at a rate of about ⅛ of an inch (3 mm) every minute. Immature sperm, known as spermatids, are stored in a long coiled tube (epididymis), which is attached to the testes. Once they have matured, they move on to the vas deferens, a tube that connects the epididymis to an ejaculatory duct. The whole process takes between 70 and 100 days. Mature sperm are either ejaculated during sex in a milky fluid called semen, or reabsorbed into the body.

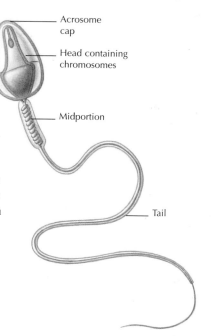

Acrosome cap

Head containing chromosomes

Midportion

Tail

GENES

Although your baby inherits 50 percent of her genes from you and 50 percent from your partner, your genes were inherited from your parents, so approximately a quarter of all your child's genes are also inherited from each of four grandparents. Genes are made up of DNA and are contained in structures known as chromosomes. At the time of conception your baby receives 46 chromosomes which exist in 23 pairs – each chromosome contains a copy of a gene from you and a matching copy from your partner. It is the combination of these genes that influence how your baby will look – they dictate hair and eye color and the shape and size of the nose and other external characteristics. Genes also provide the instructions which enable the fertilized egg to develop into a baby and are the blueprint for all the body's functions, now and in the future.

DNA consists of two chains arranged in a long spiraling ladder that "unzip" when forming new cells.

INHERITED DISORDERS

Sometimes a baby can inherit an abnormal gene or genes from either or both parents, or an abnormal gene may occur if a normal gene has become mutated during the division of cells when the sperm or the egg form. In most cases an abnormal gene won't cause a problem, but occasionally it can result in diseases such as cystic fibrosis, sickle cell disease or hemophilia. Some abnormal genes are only carried in the X chromosome and cause problems only for boys.

If you have a known history of a hereditary disease in the family you may want to consider talking to a genetic counselor to assess the chances of your baby inheriting the condition. The counselor will be able to give you the information and support you need.

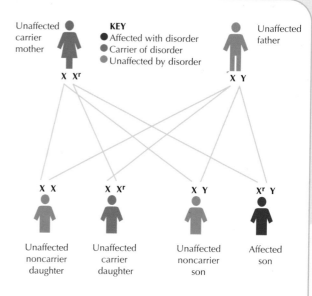

Unaffected carrier mother

X X^r

KEY
● Affected with disorder
● Carrier of disorder
● Unaffected by disorder

Unaffected father

X Y

X X
Unaffected noncarrier daughter

X X^r
Unaffected carrier daughter

X Y
Unaffected noncarrier son

X^r Y
Affected son

X = Chromosome with normal gene   Y = Chromosome without gene
X^r = Chromosome with abnormal gene

RH FACTOR

Your genes determine your blood group – A, B, AB, or O – and your Rh status – positive or negative. Known as the Rh factor, your Rh status describes whether or not you have a particular protein on the surface of your red blood cells. If the protein isn't there, you are Rh negative and this could cause complications during pregnancy. About 85 percent of people are Rh positive, but if you are one of those who is Rh negative and you are carrying a Rh positive baby (the baby gets the positive rhesus gene from his father), there is a risk of antibodies developing that can attack the baby's Rh positive blood cells, causing anemia and possibly jaundice.

You will be given a blood test to confirm your Rh status at your first prenatal check. If you are found to be Rh negative, you will be monitored throughout your pregnancy and may be given an injection of Rh immunoglobin (anti-D) at 28 and 34 weeks and within 72 hours after the birth.

 Rhesus positive gene

 Rhesus negative gene

FOLIC ACID

This is an essential B vitamin that has been shown to reduce the risk of your baby developing a neural tube defect such as spina bifida – a gap in the spine that causes damage to the central nervous system – by up to 75 percent. Ideally you should start taking a 400 mcg supplement of folic acid at least three months before you start trying to conceive and continue taking it during the first three months of pregnancy. By the end of the first trimester your baby's neural tube will be fully formed so the vulnerable period will be over. If you haven't been taking folic acid, it's not too late to start now. Also, include foods such as bread and cereal that have been fortified with folic acid, in your diet.

SMOKING

If you smoke during pregnancy the nicotine you inhale crosses the placenta and affects your baby. It will decrease blood flow to your baby, while carbon monoxide decreases the amount of oxygen this blood contains. Smoking, therefore, can lead to premature birth, low birthweight babies, and to babies being born with a cleft lip and/or palate. There is also a higher likelihood of babies developing respiratory illness such as asthma after birth. Research also suggests that there is a link between smoking in pregnancy and sudden infant death (SIDS) once the baby is born.

Smoking can also cause pregnancy complications for you and may even lead to miscarriage, placenta previa, placental abruption, and preterm rupture of the membranes.

Even though it can be very hard to do, giving up is the sensible option for both you and your baby, and it's never too late to stop. Your healthcare provider will be able to give you help and support. However, nicotine substitutes and anti-smoking medications are not suitable for use during pregnancy.

Passive smoking also can put your baby at risk, so avoid smoky atmospheres and, if your partner smokes, encourage him or her to give up, too.

ALCOHOL

It is best to avoid drinking alcohol altogether when you are trying to conceive and throughout pregnancy. This is especially important during the first trimester when your baby's major organs are forming. Even moderate drinking – having one or two drinks a day or bingeing occasionally – has been associated with miscarriage, complications during labor, and low birthweight babies. Heavy drinking can lead to fetal alcohol syndrome, which causes a range of birth defects including heart defects, mental retardation, even death. If you decide to drink during the latter stages of pregnancy you must remember that any alcohol you consume will be passed to your baby through your bloodstream. You should limit yourself to no more than two small measures of alcoholic drinks a week.

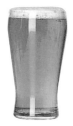 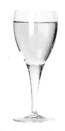 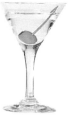

Half a pint of beer (8 fl oz or 227 ml)

A glass of wine (3 fl oz or 85 ml)

A measure of spirits (¼ fl oz or 25 ml)

An aperitif (2 fl oz or 50 ml)

MEDICATION

Don't take any over-the-counter remedies without checking with your healthcare provider. This is especially important during the first 12 weeks when your baby's major organs are forming. Some drugs, such as paracetamol, can be used in later pregnancy, but should always be taken in the correct dosage and shouldn't be used on a regular basis. Aspirin has been linked to miscarriage and neonatal heart defects; unless it has been prescribed by your doctor, it should be avoided. If you are on prescribed medication for an existing medical condition, you should discuss the dosage with your healthcare provider as soon as your pregnancy has been confirmed as it may need adjusting. It's important not to stop taking prescribed medication without taking advice because the condition it is treating could pose more risks to your pregnancy than the medication itself.

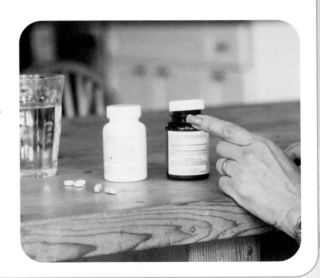

COMPLEMENTARY THERAPIES

The effects of many herbal remedies in pregnancy are unknown, so it's best to avoid them unless your healthcare provider has sanctioned their use. Essential oils used in aromatherapy can have a powerful effect, and need to be treated with caution. Ask a qualified aromatherapist for advice about oils that are safe for you to use in pregnancy. Homeopathic remedies are unlikely to cause problems to either you or your baby and can be useful in treating minor complaints but it's essential to use the right remedy, so seek advice. Reflexology and acupuncture can be successfully used to treat a number of pregnancy symptoms, but are best avoided during the first trimester – treatment later in pregnancy should always be carried out by a qualified practitioner.

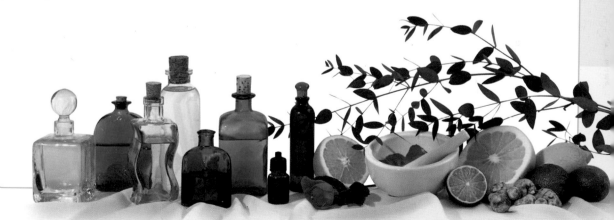

RECREATIONAL DRUGS

Taking any form of drugs during pregnancy could be dangerous for you and your baby, and this includes all types of recreational drugs. Even though there is little medical evidence on the direct effects of cannabis in pregnancy, there are studies that link the use of the drug with fetal growth retardation and low birthweight. Ecstasy has been linked to limb and heart defects in the baby and serious dehydration in the mother. Cocaine is a highly addictive drug that puts you at a higher risk of premature delivery and placental abruption as well as having a stroke, heart attack, or high blood pressure. Your baby could suffer from birth defects, neurological problems, seizures, developmental problems, and SIDS.

Heroin and other narcotics can put you and your baby at very serious risk. Moreover, your baby could be born an addict and have to go through withdrawal after the birth. Recreational drugs are a risk that can be avoided, and healthcare professionals will know how best to help any user.

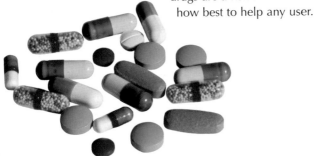

THE SEX OF YOUR BABY

Your baby's gender is dictated by your partner's sperm. Whether your baby is a girl or a boy is determined at the moment of conception by the sex chromosomes – one of the 23 pairs of chromosomes your baby gets from you and your partner. Every sperm contains either a single X (female) chromosome or a single Y (male) chromosome, while all your eggs have a chromosome containing a single X chromosome. For a girl, two X chromosomes are needed – one from you and one from your partner. For a boy, an X and Y chromosome are required, so your partner's sperm needs to contain a Y chromosome. Although there are a number of theories on how best to conceive a baby of a specific sex, none of these methods is guaranteed.

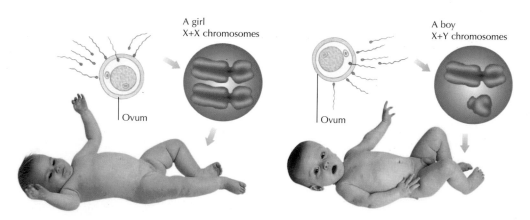

A girl
X+X chromosomes

Ovum

A boy
X+Y chromosomes

Ovum

TWINS

Non-identical twins – also known as fraternal twins – result from two eggs being fertilized by two different sperm. Each baby has its own placenta and can be of different sex. Such twins won't look any more or less alike than any other two siblings. Non-identical twins are passed down through the female and you are more likely to have twins if there is a history of them in your family. Age also plays a part, with women under 35 being more likely to conceive non-identical twins.

Identical twins are less common. They develop from the same egg which has been fertilized by a single sperm – after fertilization the egg divides into two, causing two embryos to develop. Identical twins are always the same sex and will look alike with the same hair, eye color, and blood type. The babies may or may not share the same placenta and amniotic sac, but each one will have it's own umbilical cord. Women over 35 are more likely to have identical twins.

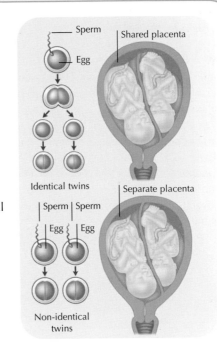

Sperm

Egg

Shared placenta

Identical twins

Separate placenta

Sperm | Sperm

Egg | Egg

Non-identical twins

TRIPLETS AND MORE

When triplets are conceived they can be identical, or a combination of identical and non-identical children. Sometimes a single egg is fertilized and then divides into three to create identical triplets. Alternatively, three individual eggs can be fertilized by different sperm to create non-identical children.

In some cases, two of the babies are created from the same egg and sperm, making identical twins, while the third baby develops from a single egg and sperm making it non-identical to the others. Quads and more can also be a mix of identical and non-identical babies. These multiple pregnancies are more common after fertility treatment when the ovaries have been stimulated to release more than one egg during the menstrual cycle, or where several "test tube" embryos are replaced in the uterus at the same time.

Here you can see two babies sharing a single sac (monochorionic twins) and a singleton triplet on his own. This is known as a mono-dichorionic triplet pregnancy.

CONCEPTION

When your partner ejaculates during intercourse literally millions of sperm are released, but only a few hundred will make it along your vagina to the fallopian tube, and only one will fertilize the waiting egg.

Sperm have to traverse the vagina, cervix, and uterus and swim out into the fallopian tubes. The fastest sperm will reach the egg in 45 minutes, the slowest take about 12 hours. Conception occurs when the head of a sperm penetrates the layers of the egg to fuse with the nucleus. A single new cell is formed, containing 46 chromosomes – 23 from each parent – with all the genetic information needed to create a new life.

Ovum being fertilized

Sperm swimming through the fallopian tube

Some sperm choose the wrong fallopian tube

The ovary

The uterus

The cervix

PREGNANCY HORMONES

Pregnancy is a time of great hormonal activity, with existing hormone levels being raised dramatically and new hormones being produced to support your pregnancy. High levels of the "pregnancy hormone" human chorionic gonadotrophin (HGC) are produced by the embryo during the first 12 weeks and it is the detection of HGC that gives a pregnancy test a positive result. The main source of other pregnancy hormones is the ovaries during the early stages and then the placenta after around 12 weeks. These hormones dictate how fast your baby grows and are responsible for changes to your breasts and body during the rest of your pregnancy.

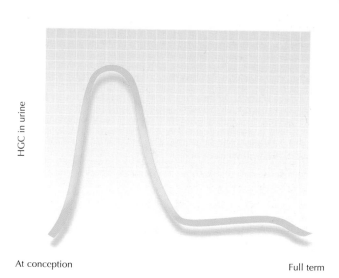

HGC in urine

At conception

Full term

ZYGOTE AND MORULA

The newly fertilized egg is called a zygote. Between 12 and 20 hours after it's been fertilized, it begins to divide in two, replicating its DNA as it does so. As it divides and subsides, the zygote is also traveling along the fallopian tube, headed toward the uterus. Hair-like feelers in the tube waft it along. The zygote divides and subdivides until it forms a solid ball the size of a pinhead. Now known as a morula, this consists of 16 to 32 cells. The morula continues dividing at 15-hour intervals, so by the time it reaches the uterus, after some 90 or so hours, it has approximately 64 cells. Of these, only a few cells will actually develop into the embryo; the rest will form the placenta and the membranes that surround the uterus.

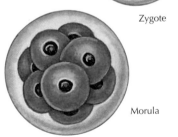

Zygote

Morula

THE THREE TRIMESTERS

Pregnancy is divided into three stages known as trimesters. Each trimester marks a major milestone in your progress and that of your baby, and you're likely to feel significantly different, both physically and emotionally, during each one. In the first trimester your body experiences the most changes as it adapts to pregnancy. During the second trimester you are likely to feel at your best as many of the early pregnancy symptoms will have passed by this stage and you will have more energy. The third and final trimester is the time when your body prepares for the birth of your baby.

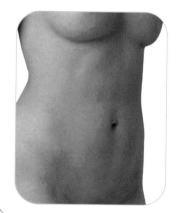 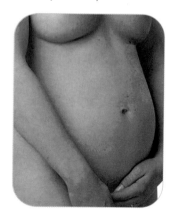 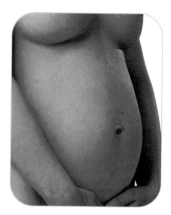

FIRST TRIMESTER

This is the first 12 weeks of pregnancy and in terms of your baby's development, a crucial period. This is when your baby develops from a single fertilized egg into a complete and complex organism. By the end of the 12th week, all your baby's major organs and body systems are formed. Miscarriage is most likely to occur during this time, so it is especially important to look after yourself now. You are likely to experience early pregnancy symptoms such as nausea and tender breasts and you may feel more emotional than normal.

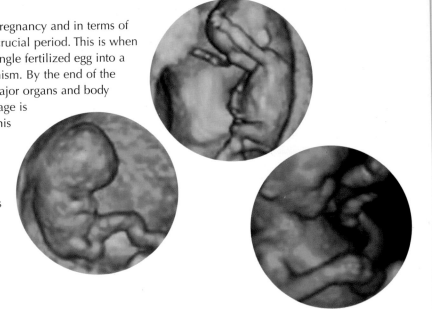

THE PLACENTA

The placenta is the amazing pregnancy organ that becomes your baby's life support system. It develops from the fertilized egg and becomes fully functional at around 12 weeks, when it starts to produce some of the hormones needed to maintain your pregnancy. The placenta is attached to the lining of the uterus and separates your baby's blood- stream from yours. In the placenta, oxygen from the air you breathe and nutrients from the food you eat flow through a fine membrane and are carried to your baby along the umbilical cord. Antibodies that protect your baby from infection pass to your baby this way, but so too do alcohol, drugs, and nicotine. Your baby's waste products are also filtered through the placenta into your bloodstream so that your body can get rid of them.

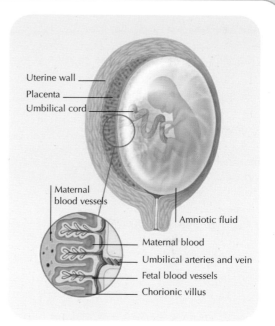

Uterine wall

Placenta

Umbilical cord

Maternal blood vessels

Amniotic fluid

Maternal blood

Umbilical arteries and vein

Fetal blood vessels

Chorionic villus

BLASTOCYST

The morula gradually develops from a solid to become a fluid-filled ball of cells, or blastocyst. Its surface consists of a single layer of large, flat cells called trophoblast cells. These later develop into the placenta. Inside the ball is a small cluster of inner cells that will become the embryo.

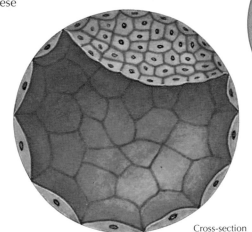

Cross-section

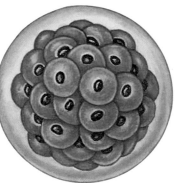

The blastocyst is less than $\frac{1}{100}$th of an inch (0.2 mm) across when it arrives in the uterus ready for implantation.

IMPLANTATION

About five to seven days after ovulation occurs, the blastocyst arrives in the uterus ready for implantation. Progesterone production is at its height. It has stimulated the rich blood vessels that supply the endometrium to grow in preparation to receive the blastocyst, which floats freely in the uterus for a few days, continuing to develop and grow.

Approximately nine days after fertilization, the blastocyst, which by now is made up of a few hundred cells, starts to attach itself to the uterine wall by means of sponge-like projections of trophoblast cells, which burrow into the endometrium. The cells grow into the chorionic villi, which will later develop into the placenta. They release enzymes that penetrate the lining of the uterus and cause tissue to break down. This provides a nourishing mix of blood cells on which it feeds. It takes about 13 days for the blastocyst to implant firmly.

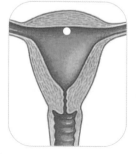

The drawing shows the usual location of implantation in the uterus.

CIRCULATION CHANGES

Soon after conception your blood volume will start to increase so that your body is able to provide adequate blood supply to your developing baby, your enlarging uterus, and the growing placenta. By the time you reach week 30, you will have 50 percent more blood circulating throughout your body. You may also notice an increase in your heartbeat as your heart works harder to circulate the extra blood volume. Your blood pressure is likely to fall during the first trimester, reaching its lowest level midway through your pregnancy. You may notice this as a feeling of dizziness when you get up suddenly, or you may even faint.

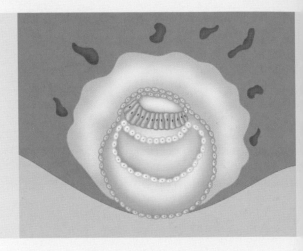

The cells within the blastocyst begin to differentiate into layers. The top (or blue) layer will become the embryo and amniotic cavity, while the lower (yellow) layer will become the yolk sac.

CONGRATULATIONS!

The fertilized egg has moved into the uterus and has probably fully implanted itself in the thickened lining, so you are now officially pregnant, even though you are unaware of this! You are unlikely to feel any differently, although some women notice their breasts beginning to feel tender even before they have missed their first menstrual period. As this is a vulnerable time for your developing baby, you should be taking extra care of yourself, eating healthily, and avoiding alcohol, cigarettes, and unprescribed drugs of any kind.

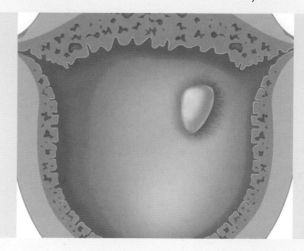

A close-up of the blastocyst burrowed deeply into the uterine wall. The rim cells of the blastocyst fuse into a tough membrane known as the chorion. This will surround and protect your developing baby.

AMNIOTIC FLUID

This is a sweet smelling, colorless liquid that fills the sac surrounding the baby in the uterus. It is made up of fluid from the placenta along with your baby's urine and lung fluid. Amniotic fluid protects your baby from temperature extremes and from being bumped or hurt as you move around. Your baby starts to swallow the fluid from about 12 weeks and continues to do so throughout pregnancy. A full-term baby may swallow as much as 1 pint in a 24-hour period. Scientists believe babies do so to aid the growth and development of the fetal digestive system. Amniotic fluid peaks at about 2 pints at 36-38 weeks and then rapidly falls off.

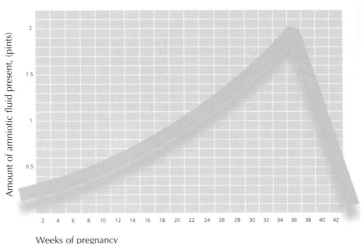

Weeks of pregnancy

UMBILICAL CORD

Sometimes referred to as the baby's "supply line," the umbilical cord is a narrow tube-like structure that connects the baby to the placenta. The cord delivers nutrients and oxygen to your baby and removes waste products. It begins to form about five weeks after conception and grows progressively longer until the 28th week of pregnancy (day 196), when it has reached a length of around 22 inches. As it gets longer the cord twists around itself and becomes coiled.

There are three blood vessels in the cord – two arteries and one vein. The vein carries oxygen-rich blood and nutrients from the placenta to the baby, while the two arteries transport waste from the baby back to the placenta.

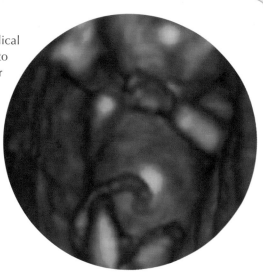

HOME PREGNANCY TEST AND PREGNANCY DATING

The home pregnancy tests that you buy over the counter work in the same way as the ones used by healthcare providers or laboratories. The tests measure the presence of the hormone human chorionic gonadotrophin (HCG) in your urine. This hormone is produced by the placenta when the fertilized egg implants in your uterus. For best results, take the test first thing in the morning, when your urine is more concentrated. Many of the tests claim to be 99 percent accurate on the day you miss your period, although to be absolutely sure you may want to wait another week.

Your pregnancy is dated from the first day of your last menstrual period (LMP) and is estimated to be around 280 days – 40 weeks, although it's quite normal for a baby to be born two weeks before or after this date. Your estimated date of delivery can be calculated by counting 280 days forward from your LMP. In reality, pregnancy is only 38 weeks long – or 266 days – because conception takes place at around the 14th day of your menstrual cycle. So, when you are described as being 12 weeks pregnant your baby will be about 10 weeks old.

Use the chart opposite to determine your expected date of delivery (EDD). Locate the date of your last menstrual period in the bold dates; your EDD will be the date below.

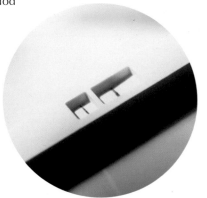

January	1	2	3	4	5	6	7	8	9	10	11	12	13	14	15	16	17	18	19	20	21	22	23	24	25	26	27	28	29	30	31
Oct/Nov	8	9	10	11	12	13	14	15	16	17	18	19	20	21	22	23	24	25	26	27	28	29	30	31	1	2	3	4	5	6	7
February	1	2	3	4	5	6	7	8	9	10	11	12	13	14	15	16	17	18	19	20	21	22	23	24	25	26	27	28			
Nov/Dec	8	9	10	11	12	13	14	15	16	17	18	19	20	21	22	23	24	25	26	27	28	29	30	1	2	3	4	5			
March	1	2	3	4	5	6	7	8	9	10	11	12	13	14	15	16	17	18	19	20	21	22	23	24	25	26	27	28	29	30	31
Dec/Jan	6	7	8	9	10	11	12	13	14	15	16	17	18	19	20	21	22	23	24	25	26	27	28	29	30	31	1	2	3	4	5
April	1	2	3	4	5	6	7	8	9	10	11	12	13	14	15	16	17	18	19	20	21	22	23	24	25	26	27	28	29	30	
Jan/Feb	6	7	8	9	10	11	12	13	14	15	16	17	18	19	20	21	22	23	24	25	26	27	28	29	30	31	1	2	3	4	
May	1	2	3	4	5	6	7	8	9	10	11	12	13	14	15	16	17	18	19	20	21	22	23	24	25	26	27	28	29	30	31
Feb/Mar	5	6	7	8	9	10	11	12	13	14	15	16	17	18	19	20	21	22	23	24	25	26	27	28	1	2	3	4	5	6	7
June	1	2	3	4	5	6	7	8	9	10	11	12	13	14	15	16	17	18	19	20	21	22	23	24	25	26	27	28	29	30	
Mar/Apr	8	9	10	11	12	13	14	15	16	17	18	19	20	21	22	23	24	25	26	27	28	29	30	31	1	2	3	4	5	6	
July	1	2	3	4	5	6	7	8	9	10	11	12	13	14	15	16	17	18	19	20	21	22	23	24	25	26	27	28	29	30	31
Apr/May	7	8	9	10	11	12	13	14	15	16	17	18	19	20	21	22	23	24	25	26	27	28	29	30	1	2	3	4	5	6	7
August	1	2	3	4	5	6	7	8	9	10	11	12	13	14	15	16	17	18	19	20	21	22	23	24	25	26	27	28	29	30	31
May/Jun	8	9	10	11	12	13	14	15	16	17	18	19	20	21	22	23	24	25	26	27	28	29	30	31	1	2	3	4	5	6	7
September	1	2	3	4	5	6	7	8	9	10	11	12	13	14	15	16	17	18	19	20	21	22	23	24	25	26	27	28	29	30	
Jun/Jul	8	9	10	11	12	13	14	15	16	17	18	19	20	21	22	23	24	25	26	27	28	29	30	1	2	3	4	5	6	7	
October	1	2	3	4	5	6	7	8	9	10	11	12	13	14	15	16	17	18	19	20	21	22	23	24	25	26	27	28	29	30	31
Jul/Aug	8	9	10	11	12	13	14	15	16	17	18	19	20	21	22	23	24	25	26	27	28	29	30	31	1	2	3	4	5	6	7
November	1	2	3	4	5	6	7	8	9	10	11	12	13	14	15	16	17	18	19	20	21	22	23	24	25	26	27	28	29	30	
Aug/Sept	8	9	10	11	12	13	14	15	16	17	18	19	20	21	22	23	24	25	26	27	28	29	30	31	1	2	3	4	5	6	
December	1	2	3	4	5	6	7	8	9	10	11	12	13	14	15	16	17	18	19	20	21	22	23	24	25	26	27	28	29	30	31
Sept/Oct	7	8	9	10	11	12	13	14	15	16	17	18	19	20	21	22	23	24	25	26	27	28	29	30	1	2	3	4	5	6	7

MISSED PERIOD?

By now you may have missed your first menstrual period and suspect that you are pregnant. You may start to experience some early pregnancy symptoms, similar to premenstrual ones, such as mood swings, heavy uncomfortable breasts, and nausea.

If you have done a pregnancy test and it was negative, you could still be pregnant – if ovulation took place later in your cycle than you thought, it may be too early to get an accurate result. Wait for a few days, and if your period still hasn't started do another test. In the meantime, avoid doing anything that could put your pregnancy at risk, such as drinking alcohol.

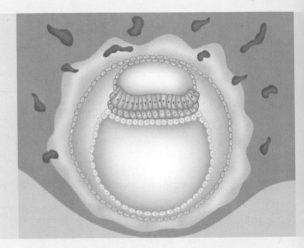

Now the embryo forms three layers: The inner or "yellow" layer (endoderm) will become the lungs, liver, digestive system, and pancreas; the middle or "pink" layer (mesoderm) the skeleton, muscles, kidneys, blood vessels, and heart; and the outer or "blue" layer (ectoderm) the nervous system, teeth, and skin.

YOUR PREGNANCY DIET

Your baby receives all its nourishment from you, therefore, it is especially important to eat healthily now that you are pregnant. You don't need additional calories until the last trimester – but equally, this is not the time to start dieting or to make any drastic changes, such as giving up meat.

Each day you should include foods from each of these food groups: Carbohydrates, fruits and vegetables, dairy products, and protein foods. It's important to avoid eating foods that are a known health hazard during pregnancy, and to ensure that you have an adequate fluid intake so that you don't become dehydrated.

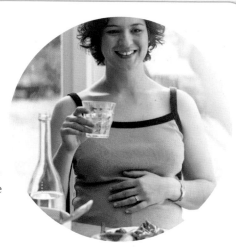

CARBOHYDRATES

Though there are broadly two types of carbohydrates, simple and complex, only the complex carbohydrates are of benefit in pregnancy. Sugars make up simple carbohydrates. Of the complex carbohydrates, unrefined carbohydrates, which are found in whole-wheat bread, pasta, breakfast cereals, brown rice, and potatoes, should form about a third of your diet. These are high-fiber foods and are good for your digestion. They will help prevent constipation, which is very common during pregnancy. Because they take longer for the body to break down, they will also help you to feel full for longer and give you energy. Often they are also rich in B vitamins. Many breakfast cereals are fortified with vitamins and minerals, including the essential pregnancy nutrient, folic acid.

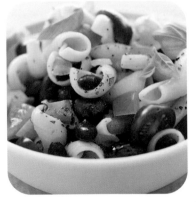

Refined cereals, used to make white bread and polished rice, are less healthy options because they contain less fiber and protein and most of the B vitamins, vitamin E and essential fatty acids are removed during their processing.

FRUITS AND VEGETABLES

Fresh fruits and vegetables should form a major part of your diet as they are high in fiber and contain many important vitamins and minerals. If you can't get fresh, then frozen and dried produce are acceptable alternatives – these will have been harvested at their best and preserved within hours so that they will have lost little of their nutritional value. Avoid over-cooking, which often destroys the vitamin content, and always take care to thoroughly wash raw fruits and vegetables before eating. To maximize your nutrient intake, you should eat a wide variety of different fruits and vegetables.

If possible, you should buy organic, as many non-organic fruits and vegetables are sprayed with pesticides and other chemicals that can be dangerous to your baby.

DAIRY PRODUCTS

Milk, cheese, and yogurts are the best sources of calcium, which is one of the most important pregnancy minerals. It helps to build your baby's bones and teeth. Eating calcium-rich foods will protect your bones, too, as your body's calcium stores are used to supply your baby's needs. An 8-oz (225-ml) glass of cow's milk will give you one-third of your daily recommended calcium requirement.

Dairy foods are also rich in B vitamins and protein. If you're concerned about putting on too much weight, choose reduced-fat versions as these retain all the minerals and water soluble vitamins of full-fat dairy products.

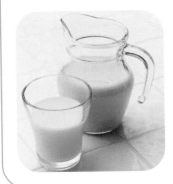

PROTEIN

You need to eat protein to help build your baby's blood cells, tissues, and organs. Protein can be found in meat, poultry, fish, eggs, and cheese, and in pulses such as peas, beans, and lentils, and nuts and seeds. These foods are also rich in vitamins and minerals and essential amino acids.

Meat, poultry, cheese, and eggs contain the best range of amino acids – plant proteins contain less, so if you're vegetarian or vegan you'll need to eat a variety of different plant-based protein, including foods made from soy, to ensure you get enough.

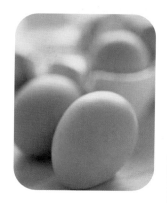

Some women worry about the hormones used in meat production and the levels of mercury found in various fish. If at all possible, buy organic and vary what you eat.

FLUIDS

It's important to keep up your fluid intake during pregnancy, so try to drink at least eight 8-oz (225 ml) glasses of fluids each day. Because pregnancy boosts your body temperature you can become dehydrated without realizing it.

Fluids are also needed to increase your blood volume, which supplies your baby with vital nutrients.

Water is the best option, but unsweetened fruit and vegetable juices, and milk are also good choices. You should limit your consumption of tea, coffee, and alcohol as these dehydrate you and can have an adverse effect on your baby.

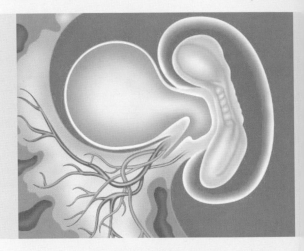

About ½ inch (3 mm) in length, your embryo is similar to the dumbbell shaped structure, right. Below his head are six pairs of segmented somites, which will form voluntary muscle, bones, and connective tissue. The embryo floats within its amniotic sac, attached to the placenta (lower left) by his umbilical cord. A yolk sac (center), supplies nutrients.

TIME TO TAKE THAT TEST

Your period is now about a week late, so if you haven't already done a pregnancy test you could do one now to confirm your pregnancy.

You may have started to experience some early symptoms such as sore breasts, tiredness, and perhaps even nausea. These early symptoms are a sign that your body is beginning to adjust to being pregnant. Of course, it's also quite natural to have none of these symptoms at this stage – but if you have, and they suddenly disappear, you should seek advice from your healthcare provider as this could be a sign of a pregnancy complication.

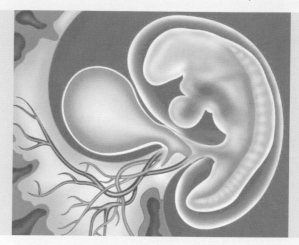

From this week, your baby's growth becomes very rapid. His neural tube will begin to close and his digestive tract starts to form. His heart, although miniscule, has one chamber and is beginning to beat on its own.

VITAMINS

Your baby needs a range of vitamins to thrive and although your body can manufacture a few of these, you need to get the rest from your food. Vitamins are quickly destroyed by exposure to heat, air, and light, and in order to maintain the supplies in food, it must be stored and cooked properly.

The most important vitamins for pregnancy are fat-soluble vitamins A, D, and E, which are stored in your body, and the water-soluble B vitamins and vitamin C, which cannot be stored and have to be supplied regularly. Although you need to take sufficient amounts of all vitamins during pregnancy, the ones mentioned here are especially important for your health and that of your growing baby. If you're unsure how to maximize your vitamin intake, talk to your healthcare provider. He or she may suggest a supplement.

MINERALS

As your body cannot manufacture minerals it has to get them from the food you eat, which is why a healthy pregnancy diet is essential to your well being and that of your baby. Iron, calcium, and zinc are particularly important as they play a big part in your baby's development. Iodine, magnesium, and selenium are also needed for a range of bodily functions, including regulating your metabolism and for the development of genetic material. All these minerals are to be found in everyday foods, so it's not difficult to achieve your recommended daily allowance. However, because nutrients are quickly lost from food, it's important to shop frequently and eat mineral sources on the same day or soon after you've bought them.

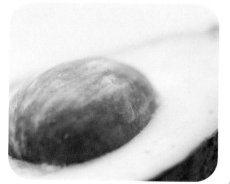

IRON AND ZINC SOURCES

Vital for new cell and hormone formation, the recommended intake of iron is 30 mg a day during pregnancy. Iron can be found in both animal- and plant-based foods. Animal sources include red meat, poultry, and fish, which contain heme-iron. Plant-based sources such as vegetables, pastas, fruits, nuts, and fortified breakfast cereals, contain non-heme iron. This form of iron is not so easily absorbed by the body as heme-iron. Vitamin C, taken alongside iron-rich foods, as in the form of orange juice, can aid its absorption, whereas tea and coffee are thought to inhibit iron absorption.

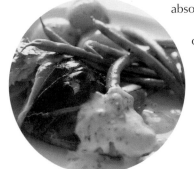

Zinc is essential for growth, immune function, and cell replication. It is present in lean red meat, eggs, canned sardines, wholegrain cereals, and dried peas and beans. You need about 11 mg daily.

FATS AND OILS

Although fats and oils should take up the smallest proportion of your daily diet, eating a small amount is good for you. Fats in vegetables, seeds, and nuts and their oils, lean meat, oily fish, and fish oils supply you with essential fatty acids, which your body can't make. Omega-3 essential fatty acids found in oily fish are important for your baby's brain and visual development. Essential fatty acids are good for you, too, as they are thought to reduce the risk of high blood pressure during pregnancy. When choosing oils, opt for mono-saturated ones like olive oil or polyunsaturated oils such as corn and safflower oils. Avoid saturated fats like butter, and those that contain hydrogenated or trans fats.

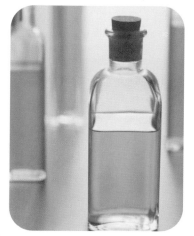

CALCIUM SOURCES

Essential for blood clotting, muscle contraction, nerve signaling, and bone and tooth growth, calcium is found in dairy products, canned fish with bones (such as salmon and sardines), tofu, and green leafy vegetables. During pregnancy, your body adapts to absorb more calcium from your food and your own calcium stores are used to supply your baby. You need at least 1000 mg daily.

It's essential that your calcium intake is high prior to and throughout pregnancy to ensure healthy bone growth in your baby. If you have a lactose intolerance, you may need a supplement.

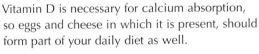

Vitamin D is necessary for calcium absorption, so eggs and cheese in which it is present, should form part of your daily diet as well.

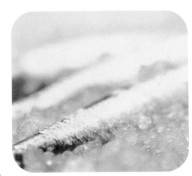

FOODS TO AVOID

Some foods should not be eaten during pregnancy because they have the potential to harm your baby. You should avoid: blue-veined cheese, unpasteurized cheese, unpasteurized sheep and goats' milk and their products, cooked foods chilled for re-heating, ready-prepared coleslaw, all types of pâté, Parma ham, hot dogs, and undercooked poultry. Undercooked eggs, and foods containing raw egg, such as home-made mayonnaise, mousses, and ice cream, should also be avoided.

Don't eat raw fish, including sushi and shellfish, and limit your intake of portions of large fish, such as swordfish and tuna, to no more than once a week.

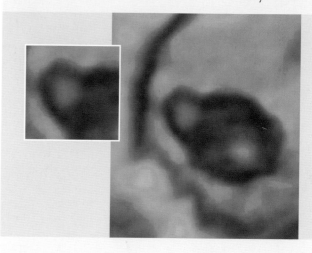

At this time, your embryo is still attached to his yolk sac, shown in close up. The placenta has not yet formed, so the yolk sac has to pass essential nutrients via a membrane to the embryo.

BREAST CHANGES AND FATIGUE

You may be experiencing some early pregnancy symptoms now. One of the most obvious will be a change in your breasts, caused by hormones stimulating the milk-producing glands. They will probably feel fuller and more tender than usual, while the veins just under the surface of the skin become more obvious as the blood supply to your breasts increases.

You may also notice that your nipples have become more prominent, while the areolas, the dark areas of skin around your nipples, become darker.

Extreme fatigue, caused by raised levels of the hormone progesterone, is also very common during these early weeks so try to get plenty of rest.

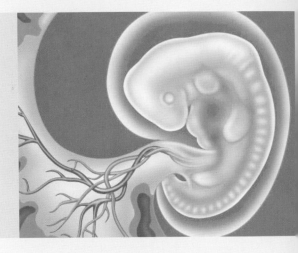

Your baby now has a disproportionately large head that bends forward from a gently curving back. His limb buds protrude more and the beginnings of hands, feet, and elbows are present. His heart is becoming a four-chambered organ and is beating at about twice the rate of your heart

CAFFEINE

Drinking excessive amounts of caffeine – over 300 mg a day – during pregnancy can lead to low birthweight and miscarriage. To be safe, you should keep your consumption to no more than two average cups of coffee, or six cups of tea, a day. Remember, too, that caffeine is also found in cola-type drinks, energy drinks, cocoa, and chocolate, so you should keep these to a minimum. Caffeine is a diuretic, drinking it will also increase your already frequent trips to the bathroom, so cutting back will benefit both you and your baby.

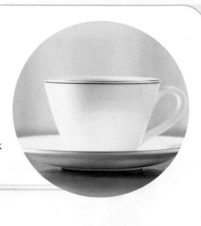

HERBAL TEAS

Herbs are drugs, so herbals teas should be treated with caution during pregnancy. If you buy herbal teas always check the ingredients to make sure they contain things that you would normally include in your diet, such as mint or orange or lemon extracts. Avoid teas that contain cohosh, pennyroyal, mugwort, and ephedra as these may have adverse effects in pregnancy. Better still, make your own using fruit juices, lemon rinds, cinnamon, and cloves along with boiled water or decaffeinated tea. Never use plants from your garden, unless you are absolutely certain you know what they are and that they're safe for use during pregnancy.

VEGETARIAN MOM-TO-BE

There is no reason why being a vegetarian should affect your pregnancy, providing you plan your diet carefully. You will need to ensure that you are getting adequate amounts of protein, iron, calcium, vitamin D, and vitamin B12. If you don't eat dairy products and eggs it will be harder for you to achieve the nutrients needed for a healthy pregnancy, and you may need to take additional supplements to boost your intake.

Discuss your diet with your healthcare provider who will be able to tell you how to boost your intake of essential nutrients and can prescribe supplements if necessary.

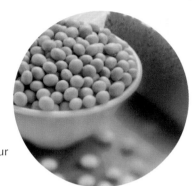

MULTIPLE PREGNANCY

Your ultrasound scan at 12 to 14 weeks will identify whether you are carrying more than one baby. If you find you are expecting twins – or more – your healthcare professionals will want to monitor your pregnancy more closely than if you were expecting a single baby. You can expect to have more frequent blood pressure and urine checks – pre-eclampsia is more common in multiple pregnancies – and to have regular scans to check on your babies' progress. You will need to have a hospital birth too, as you may require a cesarean if complications arise during the delivery of your babies.

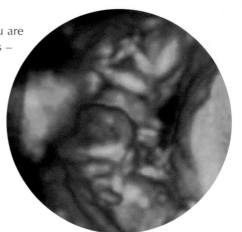

METABOLIC CHANGES

During pregnancy major changes take place as your body adapts in order to nurture your baby. All your metabolic functions are increased – including your basal metabolic rate and oxygen consumption – to provide for the demands of the baby, placenta, uterus, and your lactating breasts. Many of your internal organs are affected by these metabolic changes which is why you are likely to experience pregnancy symptoms such as nausea, constipation, indigestion, and fatigue.

You should listen carefully to your body now – for example, if your body says "rest" then you should rest.

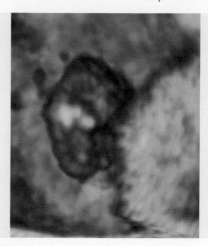

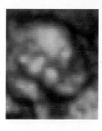

Phalangeal arches, shown in the inset, are now present. These are the structures from which elements of the face will develop.

EARLY SYMPTOMS

You may start to experience pregnancy symptoms from as early as the time of your first missed period, or you may not experience any until later in pregnancy – some women sail through pregnancy with nothing more than the occasional niggle.

Early symptoms, such as nausea and fatigue, can range from being mildly irritating to debilitating. If your symptoms seem excessive or prevent you from carrying on as normal, you should talk to your healthcare provider. The good news is that most early symptoms will have disappeared by the time you reach the second trimester.

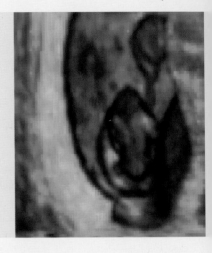

Your embryo has grown considerably and is now bigger than his yolk sac. However, this still continues to provide nourishment to him as the placental circulation has not yet been established.

LOOKING AFTER YOURSELF

You may notice changes in smell and taste, so that foods you previously enjoyed no longer appeal to you. If you are suffering from nausea don't worry too much about eating a balanced diet at the moment – it's more important to eat food that will stay down. Although your uterus is starting to swell, the enlargement can only be felt during a pelvic examination.

If you haven't already done so, you should make an appointment for your first prenatal check. These checks are important because they are designed to monitor your baby's development and to ensure that you keep healthy. They are also a good time to ask questions and to raise any concerns you may have with your caregivers.

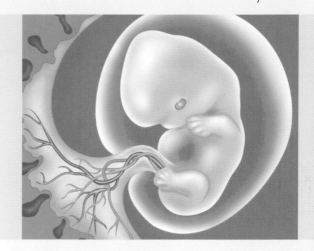

Your baby's facial features are continuing to develop. He has a rudimentary nose, with nostrils, and eyes that are open but positioned widely apart. His mouth and inner ear are developing.

NAUSEA

Although it is known as "morning sickness," nausea and/or vomiting can occur at any time of the day. Thought to be caused by the pregnancy hormone human chorionic gonadotrophin (HCG), it can start as early as week five and usually disappears – or becomes a lot less severe – by the end of the first trimester. Although unpleasant, it is harmless to you and your baby. You can help yourself by eating bland, easy-to-digest carbohydrates such as dry toast, potatoes, and rice, and by having frequent, small meals rather than three large ones each day. Ginger has been known to help combat nausea, or you could try wearing acupressure bands.

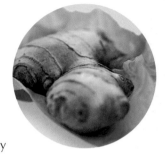

Very rarely, queasiness can get out of control, and you may not be able to keep down food or liquids. In such cases, consult your healthcare provider who will want to rule out a condition known as hyperemesis gravidarum, or excessive vomiting, which needs to be treated by hospitalization.

FATIGUE

Caused by all the physical changes that are taking place, extreme tiredness at this stage in pregnancy is normal – in fact, you may be surprised at just how exhausted you feel. Try to be realistic about what you can achieve in a day and get as much rest as you can. Going to bed early and sleeping-in on the weekends should help increase your depleted energy stores. And, although you may not feel like it, take some gentle exercise every day – you'll find that a stroll round the park, or swimming a few lengths of the pool can give you a real energy boost.

Like most early symptoms, fatigue will reduce somewhere near the end of the first trimester. However, it will reappear during the last trimester due to all the extra weight you will be carrying around.

FREQUENT URINATION

As the uterus starts to enlarge it begins to put pressure on your bladder, so you are likely to be making a lot more trips to the bathroom. An increase in the hormone progesterone also stimulates the bladder muscle so that you feel the urge to urinate, even when the bladder isn't full. This is likely to continue until the second trimester, when the uterus rises up into the abdomen, taking pressure off the bladder. The need to urinate frequently returns toward the end of pregnancy when your baby's head "engages" – drops down in the uterus – putting pressure on the bladder again.

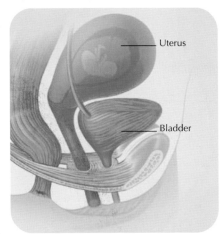

Uterus

Bladder

EXCESSIVE SALIVA

You may experience an increase in the amount of saliva you produce and notice that it has an unpleasant bitter taste. This excessive salivation is an unusual complication of pregnancy known as ptyalism. Although the cause is unknown, you are more likely to suffer from it if you have morning sickness. Ptyalism generally clears up spontaneously – usually by the third trimester. It may help to cut down on starchy foods and to eat plenty of fruit. Sucking on a piece of lemon, or chewing gum and cleaning your teeth with a minty toothpaste will help to overcome the bitter taste.

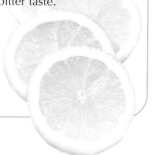

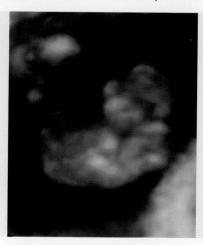

Although your baby's head is still large in proportion to his body, his trunk is longer and he's less of a C shape. Most of his internal organs have developed in a basic form.

NASAL PROBLEMS

The increase in your blood flow due to high levels of progesterone and estrogen causes the delicate mucus lining of your nasal passages to swell and soften. This can lead to an over-production of mucus and congestion, as well as occasional nose bleeds. The problem is likely to get worse as your pregnancy progresses, but will disappear after the birth.

Try to drink more fluids and use a humidifier in the home, especially in your bedroom. Vitamin C will help to strengthen your capillaries, so include plenty of citrus fruits, green vegetables, and potatoes in your diet. Annoying as this problem can be, don't use medication or nasal sprays unless they have been prescribed by your healthcare provider. Blow your nose gently to avoid bringing on bleeding.

VAGINAL DISCHARGE

It's quite common to experience an increase in vaginal discharge during pregnancy. This is due to increased mucus production and greater blood flow to the area around the vagina. As long as the discharge is white and odorless there is normally nothing to worry about. You can make yourself more comfortable by wearing panty liners to absorb it – tampons shouldn't be used during pregnancy because of the risk of infection. Try to avoid wearing tight pants, and don't use bubble bath, scented pads or toilet paper, and scented or deodorant soaps.

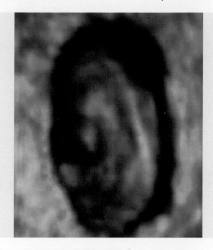

Vital Statistics

Your baby now measures ½ to ¾ inch (14 to 20 mm) from crown (the top of his head) to rump (his bottom).

9th Week of Pregnancy

It's now eight weeks since your last menstrual period. Your uterus has doubled in size and although there is no visible sign of your developing bump yet, you may notice that your clothes are starting to feel a little snug around your waist.

It's quite normal to experience unusual mood swings early in pregnancy, and you may find that you become upset more easily. Tears, anger, and occasional bouts of depression are all caused by hormonal changes in your body, together with nausea and tiredness. It's important not to let these emotions get the best of you, so talk to your partner about your feelings, or discuss them with your healthcare provider.

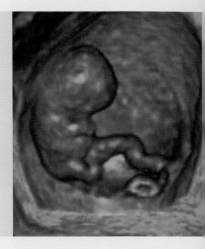

More recognizable as a baby, your embryo's head is still very large in proportion to his body. Over this week, his diaphragm will develop, and his intestines begin to move out of the umbilical cord and into his abdominal area.

BREAST CHANGES

As soon as you become pregnant your breasts start to grow – it is quite normal for your breasts to increase by as much as two bra sizes during pregnancy. You will notice that your nipples have become more prominent, and the small glands on the areolas enlarge resembling goose bumps. These changes are due to pregnancy hormones making the milk ducts grow and branch out in preparation for milk production so that you are ready to breastfeed once your baby is born. Later in pregnancy your nipples will start to secrete small amounts of colostrum, a golden yellow liquid which is your baby's first food.

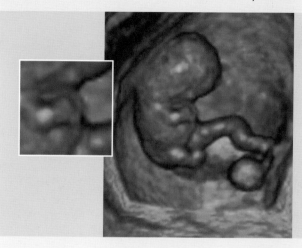

Growth of your embryo's limbs, arms, and feet is rapid. His fingers and toes are nearly complete and you can see how the hand paddles have differentiated into fingers. Nails begin to grow on his fingers and toes.

FEELING LIGHTHEADED

It's common to experience some dizziness during pregnancy and in the early weeks this is likely to occur as a result of your increased circulation. Low blood sugar levels can also contribute to lightheadedness. Include plenty of protein in your diet, and snack on fruit or whole wheat crackers when you feel the need for a quick sugar boost. Standing or sitting up too quickly affects the blood flow to your brain, which leads to dizziness. Always get up slowly so that your body has time to adjust.

Sometimes dizziness can be caused by dehydration through loss of fluids from nausea and vomiting. Make sure you increase the amount you drink.

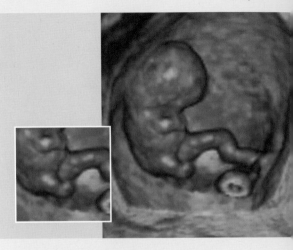

Your embryo is capable of moving both his arms and legs. The close up shows the well-developed knee joint and your baby's tiny foot – about 1/16th of an inch (2 mm) long.

FAINTING

Rarely, dizziness or lightheadedness can result in fainting. Although this won't harm your baby, it's unpleasant and it could be a sign of severe anemia, so you should tell your healthcare provider if this happens. If you start to feel faint this means that the blood flow to your brain is being temporarily reduced. You can help to stop yourself from fainting by increasing the circulation to your brain. Try lying with your feet higher than your head until the feeling passes.

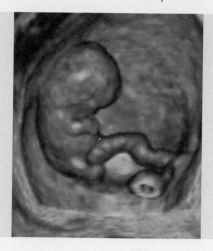

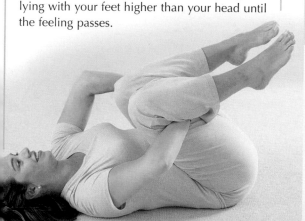

Your embryo's back is straightening, his head appears more erect, and his abdomen is tucked. He has a jaw and a nose – not readily apparent in this view! His skin is thickening and hair follciles are beginning to develop.

WEIGHT GAIN

Your healthcare provider will measure your height and weight to calculate your body mass index (BMI), a medical classification system for your body weight. Your BMI will indicate whether you are underweight, normal weight, overweight or obese at the beginning of pregnancy. If you are in the normal weight range – your BMI is between 19 and 26 – you can expect to put on between 25 and 35 lbs (11.5 to 16 kg) during pregnancy. If you are overweight or underweight you may need specialist care. Although you are likely to put on 70 percent of your additional weight during the last 20 weeks, this can vary. Don't become fanatical about your weight gain – the important thing is to ensure that your baby is developing normally.

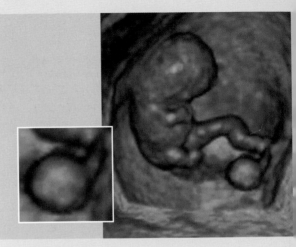

The yolk sac performs several important functions during the early weeks of life. It is involved with the transfer of nutrients and the formation of the primitive gut, and it produces blood and sex cells.

HAIR AND NAILS

Your hair growth speeds up during pregnancy so your hair is likely to become thicker and look glossier. This increase in hair growth may also lead to stray hairs appearing on your face or abdomen – remove any unwanted hair by plucking or waxing. If your hair is already dry you may find it becomes drier. If it's greasy, it may become more oily. Make sure you use mild products suitable for your hair type.

Your nails are also likely to be affected. You may find that your nails grow longer and stronger than ever before, or that they split and break more easily. Give yourself a weekly manicure and pedicure and apply moisturizing cream regularly.

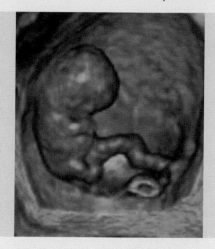

To protect his heart and eyes, your embryo's ribcage begins to close and the eyelids, which are almost fully formed, cover his eyes.

SKIN CHANGES

Increased hormone levels can leave your skin looking and feeling softer, and are partly responsible for the pregnancy "bloom" that many women experience during the second trimester. However, this increase in hormones can also lead to unwanted pimples, and even acne. You can help to control any outbreak of spots by cutting down on fats in your diet, drinking plenty of water, and taking some gentle exercise every day. Don't use over-the-counter creams without first checking with your healthcare provider, as many of these contain chemicals that could affect your baby.

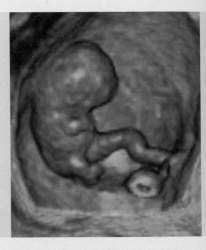

Vital Statistics

Your baby now measures about 1 inch (25 mm) from crown to rump but is still too small to merit an approximation of weight.

10th Week of Pregnancy

Your body is changing rapidly, even though there are few visible signs. You may be aware of an increase in the size of your breasts and notice that previously comfortable waistbands have becoming tighter, but it's still too soon for you to "look" pregnant.

You may find yourself unaccountably upset or irritable; this is due to the hormonal changes your body is currently experiencing.

Your gums become more susceptible to plaque and bacteria during pregnancy so you need to pay extra attention to your oral hygiene now. Brush your teeth at least twice a day and floss regularly, and arrange to have a dental check – you will need to tell your dentist that you are pregnant so that x-rays are avoided.

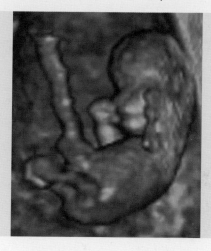

From now on, your baby is known medically as a fetus, meaning "offspring." He looks noticeably more mature than in the previous week, though his head remains large in proportion to his body. From now on an approximate weekly weight can be given.

YOUR HEALTHCARE PROVIDERS

These are medical professionals who will look after you during pregnancy and birth. Depending on where you live, you may have a choice of care – your family doctor will be able to advise you on what's available in your area. Before making any decisions, it's a good idea to also talk to friends who have recently had babies about their experiences as this will give you a more personal insight into the different types of care on offer.

Pregnancy and childbirth organizations are another useful point of contact and should be able to supply you with a list of specialist practitioners in your area.

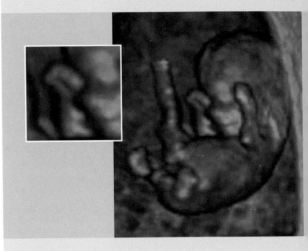

The most noticeable feature is that your baby's hand paddles have clearly defined ridges and that separate fingers and toes are emerging. The fingers develop more quickly than the toes.

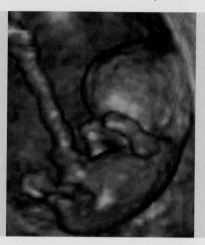

OBSTETRICIAN

This is a doctor who specializes in pregnancy, labor, and birth. An obstetrician will care for you during pregnancy and will deliver your baby in the hospital. If an assisted delivery is required, your obstetrician will be able to perform any necessary procedures, such as a cesarean. After the birth, he or she will be responsible for your care until you go home. Even if you have not chosen an obstetrician as your healthcare provider, you will be referred to one if your pregnancy is considered high risk, or there are complications during labor or birth.

Most of your baby's joints have formed, including his ankles and wrists. His feet are approximately ¹⁄₁₆th of an inch (2.5 mm) long. He is capable of a wide range of movements. This baby is shown approximating the "boxer" position.

GENERAL PRACTITIONER

This is your family doctor who can help you plan your prenatal care and may be responsible for you and your baby's medical care after the birth (unless you consult a pediatrician, a specially trained "baby doctor").

Some general practitioners are also trained in obstetrics, which means they are qualified to provide medical care for you during pregnancy and to attend the birth. If, however, complications arise during pregnancy, your family doctor will refer you to an obstetrician. If your doctor is attending you during labor and birth and a problem occurs that requires medical intervention, an obstetrician will be called in.

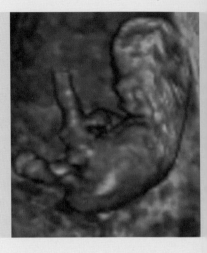

Your baby's nervous system is responsive and many of his internal organs have begun to function. His heart has attained its final shape; it now beats at 140 beats a minute.

MIDWIVES

These are people who have been specially trained to care for mothers and babies throughout pregnancy, labor, and birth. Midwives work in hospitals and they can also arrange to deliver your baby at home. If you are healthy and your pregnancy is uncomplicated, a midwife can supply all your prenatal care and will deliver your baby with the minimum of medical intervention. In the event of complications arising, a midwife can call on medical backup from other healthcare practitioners. A midwife will continue to care for you and your new baby during the first weeks after the birth.

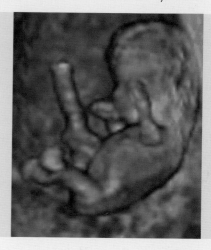

Your baby's nose and eyes are now clearly visible. However, his eyes are fused and won't open for some while. Twenty tooth buds (baby teeth) are forming in his gums.

DOULAS

Birth doulas are trained and experienced in childbirth and are able to offer help and support during labor. Their role is flexible so that they fit in with your situation and help you to achieve the type of birth you want. Doulas are not part of the medical team, but work with you as a birth partner by helping with your breathing, relaxation, movement, and positioning. After the birth your doula may follow up with postnatal visits to help you settle in at home with your new baby. Postnatal doulas specialize in offering support to new parents in the home after the birth.

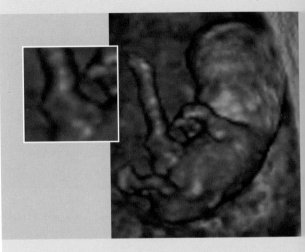

Your baby's intestines are developing in the umbilical cord; note the bulge. His stomach is developing and his kidneys are moving into their final positions in his upper abdomen.

INVOLVING YOUR PARTNER

It can be hard for your partner to feel involved with your pregnancy – especially in the early months when he can't feel or see anything.

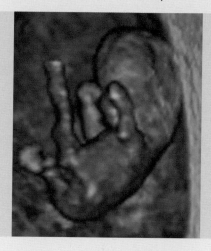

He may also be concerned about you being sick and feeling tired all the time, and feel rejected if you've stopped having sex. Talk to him about how you are feeling and encourage him to express any concerns or worries he may have. If you feel comfortable about it – and he wants to – involve him in your prenatal care and discuss the choices you have to make. Sharing your first scan together is a wonderful experience that will help make the baby seem "real" to you both.

Vital Statistics
Your baby now measures about 1⅔ inches (42 mm) from crown to rump and weighs about ⅕ ounce (5 g).

11th Week of Pregnancy

You are likely to start to experience some real weight gain now, although you will only appear a little heavier rather than pregnant. Fatigue is still a problem and you may find it difficult to sleep. If you've suffered from morning sickness it could start to lessen now, although it could still be a while before it completely disappears.

Your first prenatal appointment will be booked, so it's a good idea to write down any questions you have about your care, the type of birth you want, and how you'd like your labor to be managed. Check out your families' medical histories, too, as your healthcare provider will want to know about anything that could affect your developing baby.

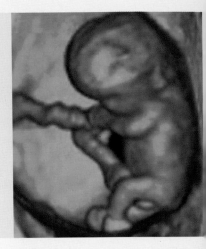

Your baby grows rapidly now. During the course of this week, he'll almost double in length. His head, however, still remains large in proportion to the rest of his body – about half his length.

FIRST PRENATAL CHECK

In this initial visit, your healthcare provider finds out everything relevant to your pregnancy. You will be asked questions about your medical history, your lifestyle, the job you do, and your personal circumstances – for example, whether you have a partner and other children. You will be given a number of tests to check that you are healthy and you may be given an ultrasound scan to confirm your due date. Sometimes, a separate appointment is made for this scan. At the end of your first prenatal check you'll be given a schedule of further visits.

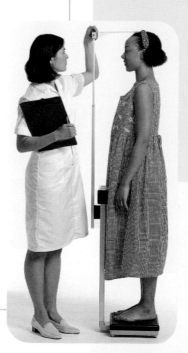

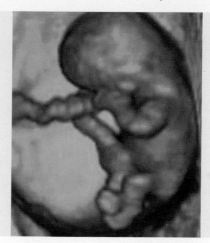

All your baby's vital organs – his brain, lungs, liver, intestines, and kidneys – are fully formed and increasing in volume.

SCHEDULE OF PRENATAL VISITS

The number of prenatal checks you have will depend on your medical needs. If your pregnancy is considered to be low risk, you will probably have monthly checks until 28 to 32 weeks. After this, you are likely to be seen every two weeks until week 36 when weekly visits are recommended. At each visit you will have your blood pressure taken and your urine will be tested. Your healthcare provider will check your baby's size and position and, from week 16 onward, will monitor your baby's heart rate.

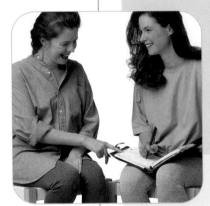

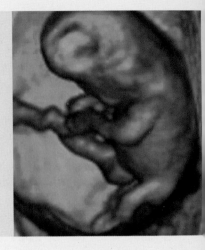

On scans, all the digits on your baby's hands and feet can be seen clearly. Fingernails start to appear.

MEDICAL HISTORY

Your healthcare provider needs to know a lot about you so that he or she can build up a complete picture of your medical history. You will be asked for information about any pre-existing medical conditions such as asthma or high blood pressure, conditions that run in either your or your partner's family, and for details of any previous pregnancies or miscarriages. Your healthcare provider will also want to know whether you smoke, drink alcohol, or use any recreational drugs, as well as how much you exercise and if your diet is healthy. The information is needed to help to ensure that you and your baby keep healthy, so it's important to be honest in the answers that you give.

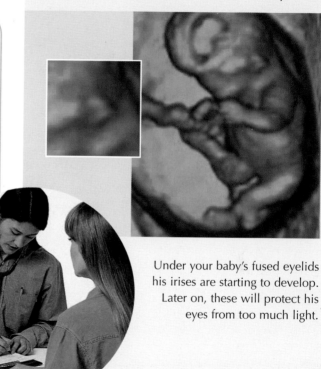

Under your baby's fused eyelids his irises are starting to develop. Later on, these will protect his eyes from too much light.

BLOOD PRESSURE

Your blood pressure is a good indicator of your overall health, so you will have it checked at each prenatal visit. There are two measurements: The higher figure (systolic) measures the blood pressure when the heart is contracting and the lower figure (diastolic) when the heart relaxes. A typical measurement is 120/70. If the reading is 140/90 or above, blood pressure is considered high. Your blood pressure is likely to decrease during the first 24 weeks of pregnancy and then return to its pre-pregnancy levels. If it continues to rise, this could be a sign of pre-eclampsia, which can be a serious pregnancy complication.

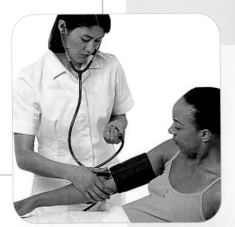

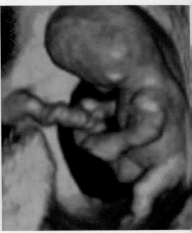

The internal development of your baby's ears is almost complete, though they are still far back on his head.

BLOOD TESTS

At your first prenatal visit you will be asked for a blood sample, which is usually taken from a vein in your arm. This sample is used to identify your blood group and Rh status, and to check your blood count to see if you are anemic. It will also be used to check for Hep B and syphilis, and your immunity to rubella (German measles).

You may be offered an HIV test; this is not compulsory, but if there is any chance you could be HIV positive, you can be given drugs during pregnancy to minimize the risk to your baby.

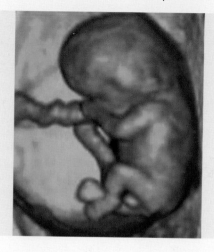

Sucking, yawning, and swallowing are all a part of your baby's repetoire of activities. He's also sufficiently grown so that he's at less risk of developing congenital abnormalities.

URINE TESTS

Your urine will be tested at each prenatal visit. You will be asked to supply a sample which will be tested during your appointment with a specially impregnated dipstick. Your healthcare professional will be looking for bacteria, glucose, and protein.

Bacteria is a sign of a kidney and urinary tract infection which, if left untreated, could cause preterm labor.

Protein could indicate an infection, or, more seriously, pre-eclampsia.

Sugar in your urine could be a sign of gestational diabetes – a form of diabetes that only occurs in pregnancy – which, if not controlled, can lead to an abnormally large baby and birth complications.

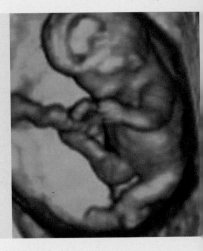

Vital Statistics
Your baby is about 1¾ to 2 inches (44 to 55 mm) long and weighs around ⅓ ounce (8 g).

12th Week of Pregnancy

As your first trimester nears its end, you may be scheduled for some diagnostic tests.

If you find that you are feeling warmer than usual and that your hands and feet are perspiring, this is due to the increase in the amount of blood being pumped around your body. You may also feel thirstier than normal – this is your body's way of telling you to drink more fluids. Try to drink at least eight 8 oz (225 ml) glasses of liquid a day, and make as many of these as possible water.

Unless nausea was a problem, you can expect to have put on around 2½ lbs (1kg) in weight by this stage in your pregnancy.

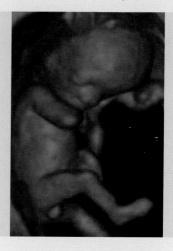

Your baby's bones begin to harden due to the laying down of calcium. The genitals take on their gender characteristics, although only an expert could say whether your baby is a boy or girl.

PRENATAL TESTS

It's natural to be concerned about prenatal testing, and the best way to allay any anxieties you may have is to make sure that you understand why the test is being carried out and what the results will reveal. Your healthcare provider will be able to explain the procedure to you and tell you whether it carries any risk for your baby. You have a choice as to whether you have a test or not, but it's important to remember that all the tests you are offered during pregnancy are designed to make sure that your baby has the best chance of being born healthy.

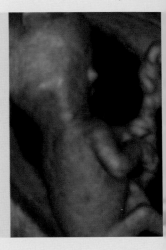

Your baby is capable of a great deal of movement, moving his torso and limbs at will. His head, though still large, is more in proportion to his trunk. Here's a good view of the back of the ear.

SCREENING TESTS

These tests can only give you the risk factor for your baby having some kind of birth defect like Down syndrome or spina bifida. The tests look for "markers" for abnormalities, such as abnormally high or low levels of chemicals like alpha-fetoprotein (AFP) or a physical characteristic such as the absence of a nose bone. Test results are classified as either low or high risk.

If you have a high-risk result, try to be positive. The reality is that a one in 250 chance of having a Down's baby is also a 249 out of 250 chance that your baby will be all right.

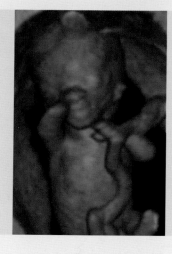

Your baby is capable of making facial gestures such as smiles and frowns at this age. Internally, his vocal chords are forming, and the pituitary gland at the base of his brain is beginning to make hormones.

ULTRASOUND SCANS

These use high-intensity sound waves to create a picture of the uterus and the baby on a computer screen. Ultrasound scanning is painless and poses no risk to either you or your baby. Your first trimester scan will be done to confirm the estimated day of delivery. The baby's measurements from crown to rump are the most accurate way of estimating the delivery date and the age of the fetus. This first scan will also identify a multiple pregnancy, and possibly diagnose certain complications and problems in pregnancy and with your fetus.

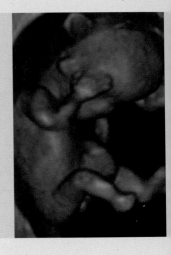

Your baby is making the most of his buoyant environment, exercising his arms and legs with a range of movements that are fluid and supple.

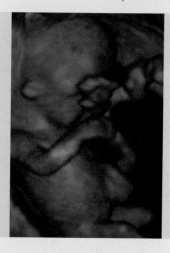

NUCHAL FOLD TRANSLUCENCY SCAN

This screening test measures the nuchal fold at the back of the baby's neck. Ultrasound is used to measure the fluid in the space, and a computer program gives an individualized risk for Down syndrome based on your age and the size of the nuchal translucency. The test is carried out at between 11 and 14 weeks of pregnancy and is considered to be 75 percent accurate. If the test is combined with a blood test, the accuracy rate rises to between 90 and 95 percent. The results from the scan are immediate, but you will have to wait a few days if you have a blood test as well.

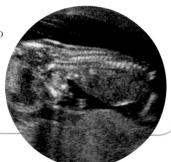

Your baby's digestive system is capable of producing the contractions that push food through his bowels and it can absorb glucose. His umbilical cord provides nourishment and gets rid of waste products produced by his rapid growth.

NASAL BONE TEST

Another screening test that can identify the risk of Down syndrome uses ultrasound to check for the presence of the baby's nasal bone. Research has shown that if the nose bone can be seen on a scan in the first trimester it is unlikely that the baby will have this chromosomal problem. The reasoning is that the noses of babies with Down's have flat bridges, with a small or poorly formed nasal bone that does not show up on an early scan. Although not widely available, this scan has recently been proven to be a good early marker for assessing the risk of Down syndrome.

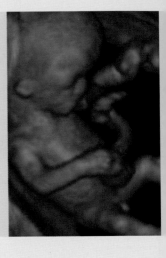

Your baby's skin is very sensitive and his reflexes are working. His vocal cords also begin to form in his larynx even though he requires air to make them vibrate and produce sounds.

EARLY PREGNANCY BLEEDING

You may experience some bleeding or spotting during the first 12 weeks of pregnancy. Any bleeding should always be reported to your doctor. Although bleeding can be a sign of miscarriage, it is more likely that you will go on to have a full-term baby.

If the blood is similar to the blood at the end of menstruation it's likely that it is caused by hormone fluctuations at the time when your menstrual period would have been due.

If the blood is bright red, you are experiencing cramps, or if you are passing clots, you may be starting to miscarry. The risk of miscarriage is much reduced once you reach the second trimester.

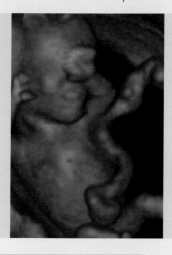

Vital Statistics

Your baby now measures about 2½ inches (63 mm) from crown to rump and weighs between ⅓ to ½ ounce (9 to 14 g).

13th Week of Pregnancy

This is the last week of your first trimester and by its end, your baby will have passed an important milestone. All his internal organs have formed. During this week, you may be scheduled for a number of diagnostic tests to check on his progress.

Your expanding uterus is now about 4 inches (10 cm) and has moved up into your abdomen, so the beginnings of a "bump" may be visible – don't worry if it isn't, some women don't show until well into the second trimester.

Any nausea is likely to have begun to fade and you may start to experience cravings for certain foods, or you may go off previously enjoyed food.

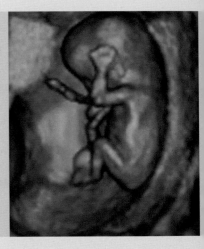

Your baby's vital organs and structures are all complete and he has arrived at a crucial stage in his development. There is now less risk of him being affected by certain drugs and infections or developing congenital abnormalities.

DIAGNOSTIC TESTS

You may be offered a diagnostic test if you have a high-risk screening test result, if you are 35 or over, or if there is a history of a genetic disease or condition in your family such as cystic fibrosis, or sickle cell disease. These tests involve analyzing DNA from your baby's cells, which are taken either from the placenta or amniotic fluid. The results usually take between seven and 14 days and are definitive. Because the tests are invasive, they carry a small risk of miscarriage.

CVS (see day 87), is normally carried out at about this time and amniocentesis at about 16 weeks' pregnancy.

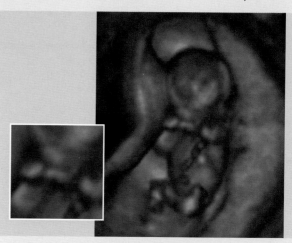

Your baby is moving constantly – though you can't feel him. He constantly alters his position in the uterus. Using the wall of the uterus as a springboard, he leaps up and down.

CVS

Chorionic Villus Sampling (CVS) is a diagnostic test used to identify chromosomal problems and genetic diseases in the baby. Fetal cells are extracted from the placenta, either through a hollow needle inserted into the abdomen or, less commonly, through a catheter inserted through the cervix. The test, which takes about five minutes to perform, is carried out at between 11 and 13 weeks. The preliminary results should be available in seven days, but you may have to wait for two weeks to get a full report. The test carries a small risk of miscarriage, but it will give you a definitive result.

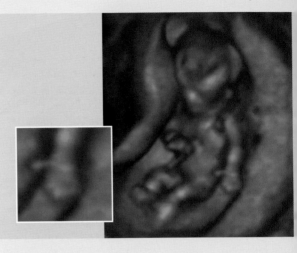

Your baby's opposable thumbs have formed. These are vital tools for all humans as they allow us to pick up, hold, and manipulate items.

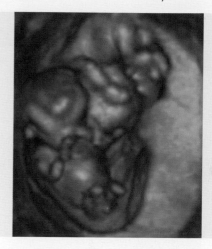

MULTIPLE PREGNANCY

Your first ultrasound scan will identify whether you are carrying more than one baby. If you find you are expecting twins – or more – your healthcare professionals will want to monitor your pregnancy more closely than if you were expecting a single baby.

You can expect to have more frequent blood pressure and urine checks – pre-eclampsia is more common in multiple pregnancies – and to have regular scans to check on your babies' progress. You will need to have a hospital birth too, as you may require a cesarean if complications arise during the delivery of your babies.

Twins begin to make contact with each other early on. One twin touching the other will elicit a reaction. But here, these twins are leading independent lives – one is awake and the other asleep.

FOOD CRAVINGS

Its very common for women to suddenly develop a passion or a violent dislike for certain foods. Spicy or pickled items, candy and chocolate, milk, fruit and fruit juices and very cold foods like ice cream are the most commonly reported cravings. Sudden aversions, however, seem to involve tea, coffee, and meat.

Some people believe that food cravings are a sign that your body is lacking in a particular nutrient, but this theory has yet to be proved. Changes in hormone levels, such as estrogen, are also thought to be responsible. Or, it could simply be that you feel your desires should be indulged now that you're pregnant.

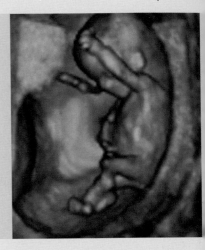

Fetuses at this age demonstrate individual variations in expression and behavior. Trained observers are able to discriminate between different babies. Your baby may also be able to sense sounds, though his ears are still not fully formed.

PREGNANCY TERMS

Health professionals often abbreviate terms when they fill out your maternity record. Ask your caregiver to explain anything you don't understand. Here are some of the most commonly used abbreviations:

BP blood pressure

Br baby is lying bottom down in the breech position

Cephalic, ceph or Vx baby's head is nearest the cervix

Cx cervix

EDD estimated date of delivery

FHH fetal heart heard

FMF fetal movement felt

Fundal height distance from the pubic bone to the top of the uterus (this is a guide to the size of the baby)

NAD no abnormality detected

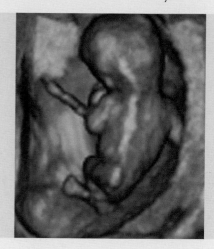

Your baby engages in a wide variety of active movements. He can jump up and down and, as you'll see on page 96, he can even grasp his feet.

PICA

This is a very rare form of craving, in which a pregnant woman has a compulsion to eat non-food substances such as ice, clay, chalk, coal, toothpaste, or even burnt matches!

Many theories have been put forward to explain this strange habit, but none has been widely accepted. What is known is that pica can interfere with the absorption of essential minerals, and if you fill up on pica substances your intake of nutritious foods is reduced. If you experience any extreme cravings, discuss them with your healthcare provider.

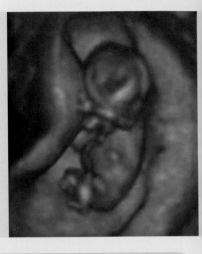

Vital Statistics
Your baby is about 3 inches (75 mm) from crown to rump and weighs approximately ⅔ ounce (20 g).

14th Week of Pregnancy

Congratulations! You have now entered your second trimester. Many of the early pregnancy symptoms will have started to fade and you should begin to feel less tired. This middle trimester is when you can really enjoy being pregnant as you're likely to be looking and feeling great. If you haven't already done so, you may want to tell your employer about your pregnancy so that you can have time off for prenatal appointments.

From this point, the risk of miscarriage is reduced by about 65 percent, and you should feel confident in your pregnancy.

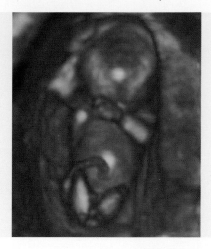

The second trimester is the time of greatest activity for your baby. He can bend, stretch, twist, kick, leap, flex, and make very complex movements with his hands.

HOSPITAL BIRTH

The majority of babies are born in the hospital. Having your baby in the hospital doesn't mean that you have to have a medicalized "high-tech" birth, unless, of course, there are complications that make an assisted delivery necessary. If everything is fine, you can choose to have your baby naturally with the minimum of medical intervention.

Being in the hospital, however, gives you access to potentially life-saving technology and specialists who can provide pain relief through epidural or spinal anesthetic. They'll be able to assist with the delivery should complications arise. This can be reassuring, especially if you are a first-time mother.

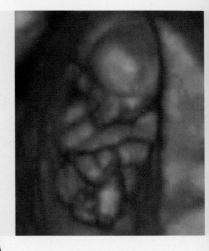

Your baby can separate his thumb from his fingers and bring his thumb to his mouth for sucking.

BIRTHING ROOMS

Some hospitals have designated rooms, which have been specially designed to allow you to give birth in a more homely environment than a sterile delivery room. These rooms often have soft lighting to create a warm atmosphere, and are equipped with birthing chairs, stools, or bean bags, which allow you to try a variety of different labor positions. They are usually large enough to accommodate you, your birth partners, and your healthcare professionals.

If you have your baby in a birthing room you will stay in the room throughout labor, birth, and recovery; some hospitals allow you to stay in the birthing room until you are ready to go home.

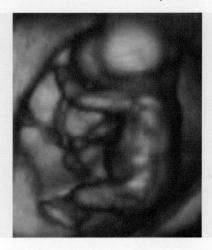

The mouth is a very sensitive organ, and thumb sucking can teach your baby about the feel of his skin, and the size and shape of his fingers.

BIRTHING CENTERS

These are usually independently run, although in some areas they are part of a hospital. Birthing centers are staffed by midwives with backup from a team of other health professionals, such as family doctors and obstetricians. You can expect family-centered care, no routine interventions, and complete control over what happens during the birth. Your prenatal care will usually be carried out at the center, too, so you'll be able to get to know the team of midwives beforehand. You will only be able to give birth at a birthing center if your health professionals consider your pregnancy to be low risk, and providing there are no complications.

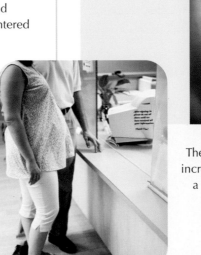

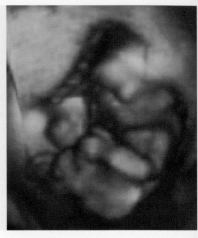

The movements your baby makes are increasingly smooth. If he's upright on a smooth surface he'll try and move forward.

HOME BIRTH

If you decide that you want to have a home birth, your healthcare provider will be able to organize this for you, providing your pregnancy isn't considered high risk. Giving birth in a relaxed, familiar environment with one's family close by is an attractive option for some women.

You will be looked after by midwives, who will help you to give birth as naturally as possible. If at any stage you change your mind, or an unforeseen complication arises, you can still be transferred to the hospital. Research shows that a home birth can be as safe as a hospital birth for healthy women at low risk.

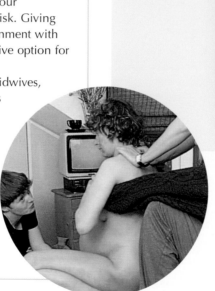

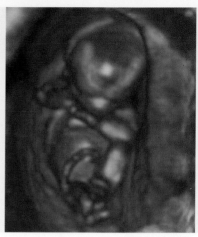

Your baby is able to bend his knees and his hands at the wrists.

ACTIVE BIRTH

Having an "active" birth means that you take an active role rather than a passive one during labor and birth. Active birth classes will teach you how to use breathing, different positions, birth aids, massage, water, and complementary therapies to help you during labor, and also inform you when and how to use medical interventions should you need them. Being active during labor means you are not confined to bed, so that contractions are more effective, while being upright allows you to achieve the best position for birth. You can have an active birth in hospital, a birthing center, or at home.

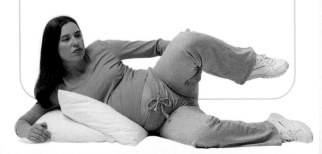

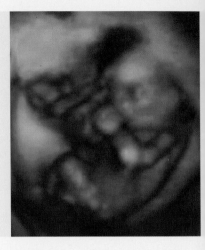

Your baby has acquired several reflexes: If his palms are touched, he will close his fingers; if the soles of his feet are stimulated, his toes will curl down.

NATURAL BIRTH

This means giving birth as naturally as possible without drugs, or any medical intervention – unless it becomes necessary for your safety or the safety of your baby.

A natural birth gives you a great deal of control over how your labor and birth are managed – for example, whether labor is induced or the membranes are artificially ruptured. You can choose how mobile you want to be, which birth position you want to try, and what labor aids to use. Instead of drugs, you use relaxation and breathing techniques to help you cope with contractions.

You can have a natural birth at a birth center or at home, but if you have your baby in the hospital, you'll need to check its policy on natural birth.

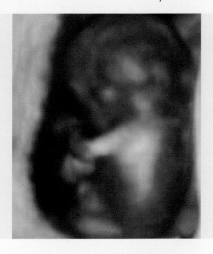

Vital Statistics
Your baby is about 3¼ to 4 inches (80 to 104 mm) from crown to rump and weighs just under an ounce (25 g).

15th Week of Pregnancy

You should be over the worst of any early pregnancy symptoms by this week, and you are likely to be feeling a lot better and more energetic than before.

You may begin to notice a change in the appearance of your skin. Freckles, moles, and nipples are probably darkening in color as your skin becomes more deeply pigmented. Sun can intensify discoloration; make sure you use a sunblock with at least an SPF of 15. Also, you may have to adapt your daily cleansing and moisturizing routines to accommodate any changes, making sure that you use hypo-allergenic products suitable for your skin type.

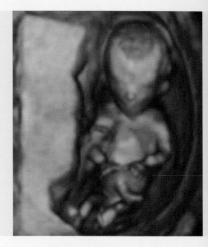

More bone is being deposited on your baby's skeleton, making it easier for him to bend his arms at the wrist and elbow. He can make varied movements with his hands.

DENTAL CARE

It's especially important to look after your teeth now as the pregnancy hormones circulating in your body can cause your gums to swell, making them susceptible to plaque and bacteria, and more likely to bleed when you brush and floss. Use a soft-bristled toothbrush and floss gently and then massage your gums to improve the blood circulation. Chewing sugar-free gum will also help prevent plaque building up on your teeth. You should see your dentist every six months for a check up. If your dentist feels you need treatment, you may be advised to wait until after you've had your baby.

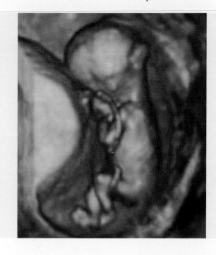

The very small bones of your baby's inner ear have begun to harden. Here, you can see that the developing external ear is nearing its final position on the head.

105

DENTAL FILLINGS

Many experts believe that amalgam fillings should not be inserted or removed in pregnancy because they contain mercury, which poses a slight risk to an unborn baby. If you need a filling while you are pregnant, you should discuss your options with your dentist. You may be offered a non-amalgam one, or a temporary one, which can be replaced after you've had your baby. Don't worry if you already have amalgam fillings – there is no evidence to suggest that ones already in place have any affect on an unborn baby.

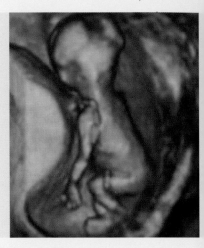

Although its very hard to discern, a downy type of extra-fine hair is starting to cover your baby's skin. This will help him regulate his body temperature.

SKIN MOISTURIZING

As your abdomen and breasts grow the skin in these areas will become stretched, making it feel dry and itchy. Massaging your abdomen and breasts – avoiding the nipples – with a light aqueous cream or oil will keep your skin moisturized and help soothe any itching. Your skin will absorb more moisture when it is wet so it's best to apply any cream or oil after washing, while your skin is still damp. You'll find that gently massaging moisturizer into your abdomen is also a great way of communicating with your baby.

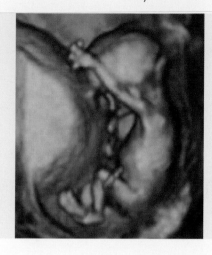

Your baby's skin is still wafer thin, and you can easily see his ribs and possibly his blood vessels.

STRETCH MARKS

These are red or purple lines that commonly appear on the lower abdomen, thighs, hips, buttocks, and breasts, which are caused by a sudden increase in your weight. If you put on a lot of weight in a short time, your skin doesn't have the chance to adapt. It stretches and the collagen in the skin separates, causing visible lines.

There is little you can do to prevent stretch marks, although keeping your skin well-hydrated and healthy through regular moisturizing and by drinking plenty of water will allow it to stretch more easily. Applying pure vitamin E oil may help reduce visible marks. Stretch marks fade over time to a silver sheen.

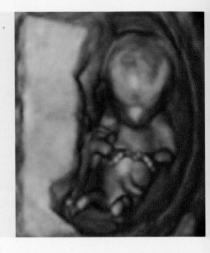

Your baby's arms are now sufficiently long so he can touch his hands together, but his brain hasn't developed sufficiently so that he "knows" he is touching another part of his body.

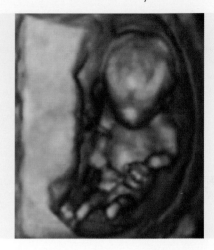

CHLOASMA

Also known as "the mask of pregnancy," chloasma is a patch of pigmentation which appears on the face – usually across the forehead, cheeks, nose, and chin. If you are fair skinned, the pigmentation will be dark; if you're dark skinned, it will be lighter than your normal skin color. Use concealer to help hide these marks and apply a UV sunscreen before going outside to prevent any further increase in the pigmentation. Chloasma is caused by hormonal influences on the skin pigmentation cells during pregnancy and will gradually disappear after the birth when your hormones return to their pre-pregnancy levels.

Your baby is acquiring eyelashes and head hair and his eyelids are fused closed. However, he is capable of demonstrating a wide array of facial expressions.

LINEA NEGRA

As your pregnancy progresses, you may notice a brownish line running down the middle of your abdomen from your navel to the pubic bone. This line has always been there, but you may not have noticed it before because it was the same color as your skin. During pregnancy the line, known as the linea negra, becomes darker. If you're fair skinned, it may hardly be noticeable, but on dark skin it can appear quite prominent. Like most pigmentation changes that occur during pregnancy, this will gradually disappear once your baby has been born.

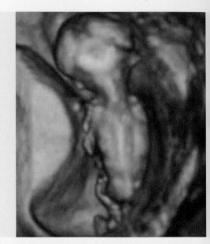

Vital Statistics

Your baby now measures between 4 and 4½ inches (104 to 114 mm) from crown to rump and weighs about 1¾ ounces (50 g).

16th Week of Pregnancy

You could be feeling in an in-between stage now as your normal clothes become uncomfortable but you're not really big enough for maternity wear. You may want to invest in some tops in the next size up and pants or skirts with elasticated waists that will see you through the next few weeks until you are ready to buy maternity clothes.

The second trimester is the best time for a vacation; you're likely to be feeling better now than at any other time of your pregnancy. Plan to take your holiday before you reach 28 weeks, as some airlines won't allow you to fly after this time.

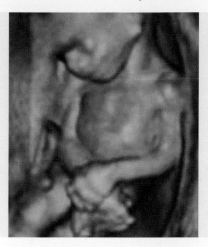

The formation of your baby's arms and legs is complete and now his legs are longer than his arms. All his joints "work" and he can move everything. The bones that he has are becoming harder and retaining calcium.

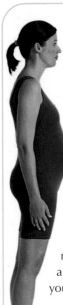

YOUR PREGNANCY POSTURE

As your pregnancy progresses, the uterus expands, rising up into your abdomen so that the weight of your baby tips your pelvis forward, shifting your center of gravity. Your natural tendency to compensate for this will be to lean back slightly, which puts pressure on your lower spine, causing backache. The increased weight of your breasts can also affect your upper back, leading to aches and pains in your upper body. You will need to take extra care of your back and make a conscious effort to keep your posture balanced.

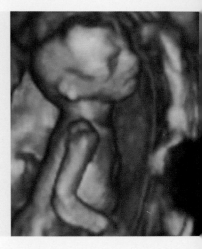

Your baby's nervous system is operating and his muscles respond to stimulation from his brain so he can coordinate his movements.

ABDOMINAL MUSCLES

These are the muscles that support your expanding uterus and help to push your baby out during the second stage of labor. During pregnancy, production of the hormone relaxin allows your abdominal muscles to stretch in all directions to accommodate your growing baby. Because your waistline can increase by up to 20 inches, these muscles have to lengthen and stretch away from their central position. This opening out of the muscle bands isn't painful so you are unlikely to be aware of it.

Occasionally, the muscles that run down the middle of your abdomen, the rectus abdominus, are too tight to stretch over the expanded uterus so they separate to form a slight gap. This is a painless condition known as rectus diastasis.

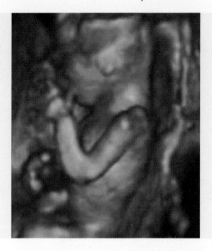

Babies are commonly seen bringing their thumbs close to their mouths and will suck them when the opportunities arise.

NUTRIENT-PACKED SNACKS

If you are finding it hard to eat three meals a day, don't be tempted to miss a meal. Instead, eat smaller amounts at mealtimes and fill up in between with healthy snacks.

Try snacking on fresh or dried fruit, raw vegetables, yogurts, and smoothies, and carry small packs of raisins or dried apricots in your bag to eat when you feel the need for something sweet.

Although cookies and candy are tempting, they only contain empty calories, which have no nutritional value. The occasional treat won't do you any harm, but they should be kept to a minimum.

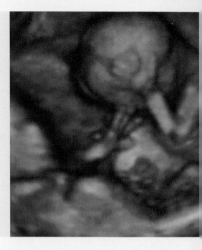

Twins interact together from an early age. Contact begins at about 12 weeks of pregnancy and generally there is an action-reaction sequence. More complex behavior, of longer-lasting contacts, begins as the brain develops.

WORK HAZARDS

Your employer is responsible for your health and safety in the workplace. If you are worried that your job entails risks, you should discuss your concerns with your health and safety officer. If you work in an office, you are unlikely to be in any danger from the equipment you use. However, if you work with chemicals or other biological agents, or use machinery that could put you at risk, your employer will need to find an alternative job for you.

If you have to lift and carry items, make sure you know how to lift correctly and avoid lifting or carrying heavy objects.

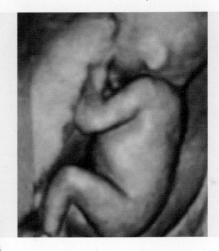

Your baby's immune system can now produce antibodies, although he is dependent on your antibodies, which cross the placenta.

HOME HAZARDS

Most household cleaners won't affect your baby, but try to avoid using products with strong fumes, such as oven cleaners, unless the room is well ventilated. Repeated exposure to chemical insecticides can be harmful; use environmentally friendly products, which won't pose a risk to your baby. Some older paints contain lead so don't strip old paint or use latex paints, which may contain mercury. if you want to paint the nursery, get someone else to do it, using water-based paints.

Cat feces can cause toxoplasmosis; wear gloves when changing the litter box and wash your hands afterward. You should wear gloves, too, when you are gardening.

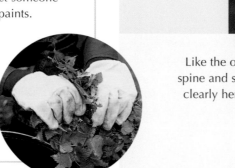

Like the other bones in his body, those of his spine and shoulder blades, which can be seen clearly here, are taking on more calcium and becoming harder.

FOOD HAZARDS

Because of the risk of infection from bacteria found in food you need to take extra care when preparing meals.

Make sure that eggs and meat are well cooked and fruits, vegetables, and salads are well washed. Always wash your hands and work surfaces before and after preparing food, and wash all cooking utensils thoroughly after use.

Never refreeze food once it has been thawed and don't eat anything that is past its "sell by" date. Keep raw meat and poultry on the bottom shelf of the refrigerator and store raw and cooked foods separately.

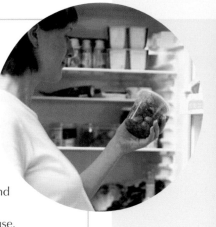

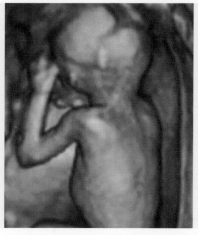

Vital Statistics

Your baby now measures about 4⅔ inches (116 mm) from crown to rump and weighs approximately 2¾ ounces (80 g).

17th Week of Pregnancy

Your breasts are continuing to grow and they may be feeling more tender. If you haven't bought yourself a bigger bra yet, you may need to go and get yourself measured for a larger size now.

Because your body is holding more water than normal you may start to experience slight swelling in your hands and feet, especially at the end of the day. Try wearing low-heeled, comfortable shoes and sit with your feet up whenever you can to reduce any swelling in your feet.

As there is a slight chance that swelling could be a sign of pre-eclampsia, you should tell your healthcare provider about it at your next prenatal check.

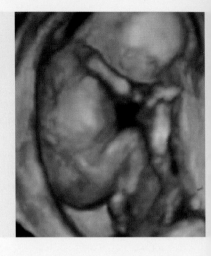

Your baby's heart is pumping as much as 25 quarts (24 liters) of blood a day and his circulatory and urinary systems are working perfectly.

MATERNITY CLOTHES

When it comes to buying maternity clothes you'll be spoilt for choice. But don't rush out too soon to buy your maternity wardrobe – you've still got a long way to go and you don't want to be sick of your clothes before you reach the end of pregnancy.

Because of the wide range available, you don't have to change your image just because you are pregnant. Look for garments that suit your normal style, in easy-care fabrics that will continue to look good as your bump increases in size.

You can buy maternity clothes in department stores, specialized maternity wear shops, through mail order and from second-hand shops. Generally, maternity clothes are more expensive than conventional garments.

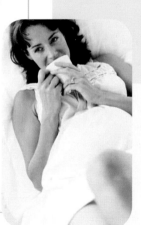

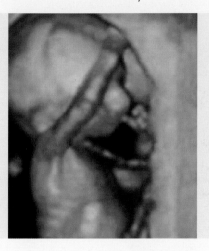

Your baby can do a lot with his hands, including putting his fingers into his mouth. His fingers are very well developed.

WARDROBE ESSENTIALS

A few well-chosen items that you can mix and match should see you through until after the baby's born. If you need to look smart for work, a jacket with a matching skirt and trousers and a selection of tops will give you a variety of looks.

A pair of black, straight-legged trousers can be dressed up or down by teaming them with a stylish top or a casual T-shirt.

Complete your wardrobe with a bias cut dress, a skirt, a few T-shirts and a stretchy cardigan, and some sweat pants for lounging around in at home. You'll also need underwear and some comfortable shoes.

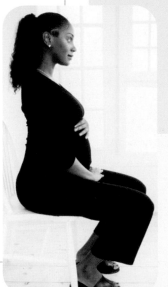

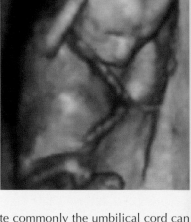

Quite commonly the umbilical cord can be seen draped around a baby's neck. This is not a cause for worry as it is too tough to become knotted.

BRAS

Although you probably won't need a maternity bra until later in pregnancy, you will need to wear a well-fitting support bra with wide comfortable straps as soon as your breasts start to increase in size. Ideally, you should have your breasts measured by a professional fitter who will then be able to advise you on the best style for your shape and size. You can expect to increase by a bra size and at least two cup sizes over the nine months. By around week 36 you may want to be fitted for a nursing bra, suitable for breastfeeding later. If your breasts are uncomfortable at night wearing a lightweight sleep bra will help.

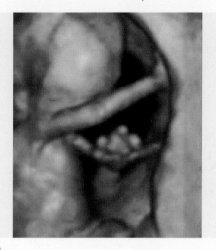

Lacking subcutaneous fat, your baby is still quite thin.

121

TIGHTS AND STOCKINGS

It's important not to wear anything that may restrict your blood flow, as this could lead to varicose veins. Don't wear tights or knee-high stockings with tight elasticated tops. Try maternity tights, which have an extra panel in front that fits over the bump and a soft waistband that sits above it.

If you suffer from aching feet and legs or varicose veins maternity support tights, which offer light, medium, or firm support will make you feel more comfortable. You may find it helpful to put them on in the morning before you get out of bed.

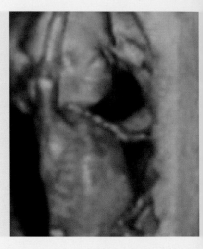

Your baby's eyes remain closed, but underneath his eyelids his eyes have grown larger. He has eyebrows and eyelashes.

SHOES

Avoid high heels or flat shoes that will throw your posture out and cause backache. Instead, wear low-heeled shoes that you can slip on and off easily – lace-up and buckle styles may be all right now, but will become difficult to do up later in pregnancy.

Shoes should be made from a material that allows your skin to breathe, as your feet are likely to be sweatier than normal. It's good idea to alternate the shoes you wear each day so that they have a chance to dry out before you wear them again. If your feet swell, you may find that a larger shoe size is more comfortable.

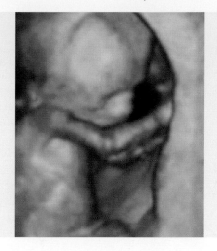

Your baby practices respiratory movements now; amniotic fluid passes into and out of the air passages in the lungs.

SPORTS WEAR

Whatever exercise regime you follow, make sure that you wear appropriate clothing and footwear. You are likely to get hotter than usual, so wear layers that can be discarded as you warm up. You'll also need a good sports bra for comfort and to give your breasts additional support while you exercise.

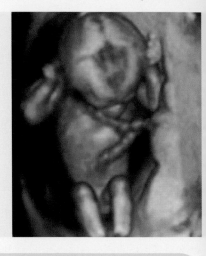

Choose cotton socks rather than socks made from synthetic material. The former will absorb moisture, the latter will prevent your feet from breathing. It's important that your sports shoes give your feet and ankles adequate support as this will assist you in maintaining your balance.

Vital Statistics

Your baby measures about 4½ to 5 inches (11 to 12 cm) from crown to rump and weighs approximately 3½ ounces (100 g).

18th Week of Pregnancy

You may have noticed that your trips to the bathroom have become less frequent. This is because the uterus moves up into your abdomen as your baby gets bigger so there is less pressure on your bladder.

Your heart rate has increased its output and this extra volume of blood can make the veins in your arms, legs, and breasts more noticeable. It can also cause minor nosebleeds and you may have some nasal congestion. Don't use over-the-counter medication to try and clear the problem, as these may not be suitable for use in pregnancy. Instead, talk to your healthcare provider, who will be able to advise you on the best treatment.

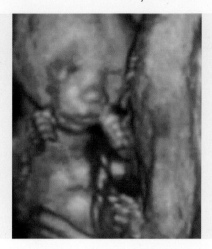

At around this time, your baby's brain is developing the neural pathways that will enable him to begin to sense the other parts of his body.

EXERCISE

Regular exercise will improve your fitness so that you are better able to cope with pregnancy, labor, and birth; it will also help you regain your shape more quickly after you've had your baby. But some medical conditions mean that you need to take extra care when exercising, or may even mean you shouldn't exercise at all, so check with your healthcare provider before you begin or continue with an existing exercise program.

Now is not the time to take part in competitive sports such as racquet and contact sports, or to do high-impact aerobics or jogging. Choose exercise such as walking, swimming, and yoga, which can be done at a gentle, rhythmical pace that can easily be adapted to suit each stage of your pregnancy, or enroll in a prenatal exercise class.

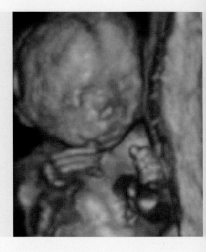

Your baby continues to exercise his hands. He can make his hand into a fist, and open and close it.

WARMING UP AND COOLING DOWN

Whatever form of exercise you do – even if it's gentle, such as walking – it's important to warm up before you begin and allow a cooling down period when you've finished. Warming up for between five and ten minutes will increase your blood flow and warm your muscles so that they stretch more easily.

A gentle cooling-down period, which stretches each muscle group in turn, followed by relaxation or deep breathing exercises, will help your body to return to normal once you've finished exercising.

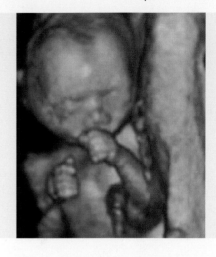

Pads have formed on your baby's fingertips and toes, and the unique swirls and whorls that will be his fingerprints begin to appear.

PREGNANCY STRETCHES

Stretching is a good way to exercise all your muscles and is especially good for pregnancy as many of the exercises can be done sitting or standing. Stretching will improve your posture and help prevent backache, it can also help relieve common complaints such as cramp in the legs and feet.

Always warm-up your muscles with gentle exercise such as walking on the spot or stationary cycling before you begin, and avoid big, energetic movements, which could over-stretch your muscles. Include some stretches in your warm-up or cool-down routines when you're doing other forms of exercise.

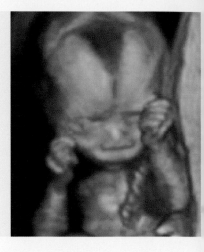

Inside your baby's fast-growing lungs, tiny air sacs called alveoli are beginning to develop.

SEATED STRETCHES

These can be done throughout pregnancy, even during the third trimester, when your bump can make exercise more difficult. This seated chest stretch will stretch and lengthen your chest muscles, which will improve your posture.

Sit on the floor with your legs crossed. Rest your hands on your buttocks, tighten your abdominal muscles to lift your baby, and sit tall. Keeping your abdominals tight, lift your chest and draw your elbows back, squeezing your shoulder blades together – remember to keep breathing. You should feel the stretch across your chest and the front of your shoulders.

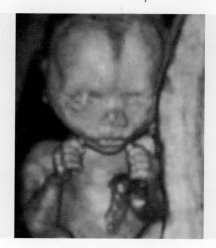

Your baby's urinary system is fully operative. Undigested debris from swallowed amniotic fluid is accumulating in his lower bowel.

129

STANDING STRETCHES

Most stretches can be done standing up although you may find it helpful to use the back of a chair to help you balance. This quadriceps stretch will stretch and lengthen the muscles at the front of your thighs, which often become tight during pregnancy.

Stand with your feet hip-width apart and rest your hand on the back of a chair. Flex your left knee slightly and lift your right knee in front of you, holding your ankle at the front. Move your right knee back until it is directly under your hip and lift up through the foot. Tilt your pelvis forward slightly and keep your abdominals tight. Hold until you feel the stretch at the front of your thigh. Repeat with your left leg.

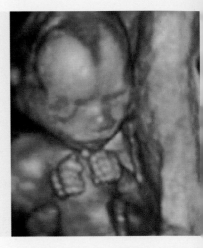

Brown fat, which will help your baby to regulate his body heat once he's born, is beginning to form. This also gives him energy. The uterus, of course, seen on the right, is a safe, warm environment for him.

ABDOMINAL EXERCISE

Strong abdominal muscles will not only help you maintain good posture, but will also make it easier to push the baby out during delivery. Although previously you will have done abdominal exercises lying on your back, after the fourth month of pregnancy the uterus presses on blood vessels and can restrict the flow of blood to your heart and baby so you'll need to adapt the exercises so that you can do them sitting, standing, or lying on your side.

Sit on a chair and place you hands by your side or behind your head. Slowly curl your body toward your knees, contracting your abdominal muscles. Relax and repeat as many times as you can without tiring yourself.

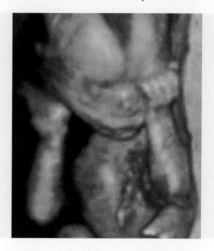

Vital Statistics

Your baby is about 5½ inches (14 cm) from crown to rump and weighs approximately 5¼ ounces (147 g).

19th Week of Pregnancy

You may be able to feel your baby move this week. These first movements are hard to describe, but you may feel them as butterflies in your stomach, or a slight bubbling feeling, rather like gas. Don't worry if you haven't felt your baby yet – it's quite normal not to feel anything for another two or three weeks.

Your healthcare provider will be able to hear your baby's heartbeat using a Doppler probe. At your next prenatal appointment, ask if you can listen to it, too. Your growing bump may start to affect your balance, so take care when you are out and about, and avoid climbing on chairs or stepladders now.

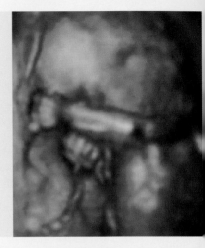

Vernix caseosa, a thick, white, greasy substance, is being secreted by glands in your baby's skin. This will act as a waterproof barrier to protect him.

PELVIC FLOOR EXERCISES

Of all the exercises you do during pregnancy, these are the most important. Your pelvic floor muscles support the uterus, bladder, and bowel, and they need to be kept toned to support your baby's weight and to prevent incontinence after the birth. You can identify these muscles by briefly stopping the flow of urine midstream when you go to the bathroom. You can exercise these muscles anywhere – sitting watching TV, standing in line, or while you are washing dishes. Simply squeeze these muscles, drawing them in as far as you can, hold for a count of five, and gradually relax.

Don't do these exercises while urinating; this could cause a urinary tract infection.

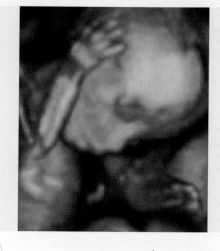

Pelvic floor muscles contracted

Although your baby's eyes remain closed to protect them, they are now in their correct position.

WALKING

This a relatively risk-free form of exercise which can be done anywhere – although you are likely to enjoy it more if you walk in a park or the countryside. Walking will not only keep you fit, but can also help to reduce swelling of the feet and ankles and may lessen the discomfort of varicose veins. It's also a good way to relieve stress and clear the mind.

How much you walk will depend on your level of fitness, but try to achieve a brisk 20- to 30-minute walk each day. Pay particular attention to your posture when you're walking and wear comfortable shoes and a jacket or sweater you can take off if you become hot. Safeguard your muscles by allowing time for a warm up and cool down.

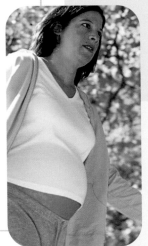

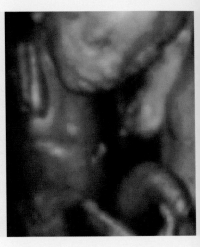

The debris accumulating in your baby's lower bowel is a paste-like material called meconium. It will form part of your baby's first bowel movement.

YOGA

Combining breathing and relaxation techniques with stretching, strengthening, and balancing exercises, yoga is the ideal exercise choice for pregnancy. Yoga postures help to strengthen the heart muscles and increase lung elasticity, making them work more efficiently. Yoga will also help to raise your energy levels and improve your circulation and digestion.

Regular yoga practice encourages body awareness and helps you to recognize what your body needs. Ideally, you should go to a prenatal yoga class where the exercises are tailored to pregnancy. If you already attend a yoga class, make sure that your instructor knows you are pregnant, as not all the exercises are safe for pregnancy.

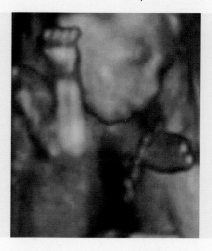

Your baby's gut is starting to produce gastric juices that help him to absorb amniotic fluid and pass it into his circulation.

PILATES

This is a form of exercise that combines flexibility and strength training with body awareness and breathing. All the exercises are based around your central core – your abdominals and pelvic floor muscles. Pilates can be useful in strengthening these muscles, although as your pregnancy progresses you may find it becomes more difficult to tighten and hold them. Some Pilates exercises are done lying on your front or back – but these positions are not suitable from mid-pregnancy onward.

If you want to do Pilates, look for classes specially designed for pregnant women, where the instructor will know how to adapt the exercises for different stages of pregnancy.

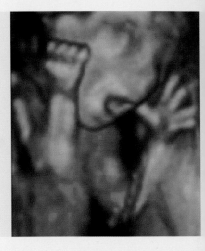

Babies in the uterus demonstrate a wide variety of facial expressions. Your baby, like this one, might be seen looking as though he is complaining, but, more likely, he is getting ready for some finger sucking.

GOING TO THE GYM

If you were working out at the gym prior to pregnancy, and your healthcare provider agrees, there is no reason why you shouldn't continue with your normal routine. You may have to adjust the resistance as your pregnancy progresses, and you must avoid any machines that require you to lay on your back such as the bench press. Later in pregnancy, you may find that your bump gets in the way so that sitting on the machines is uncomfortable. You can still work out using free weights, but don't overdo things. It's really important not to hold your breath or bear down when you are weight training.

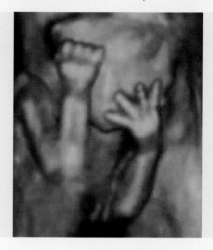

Myelin, a fatty nerve coating, is being produced. This insulates nerves and allows for a smooth, rapid exchange of information that allows your baby to perform more skilful movements.

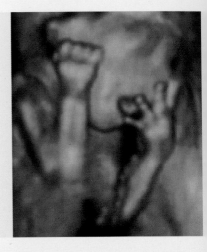

EXERCISING SAFELY

There are certain precautions you'll need to take when you exercise to ensure that you and your baby are not put at risk.

Don't exercise if you are fatigued, especially in late pregnancy. Make sure that you don't become overheated; never exercise vigorously in a hot, humid atmosphere or if you have a fever. Drink plenty of water before, during, and after exercise to prevent dehydration. Eat regularly and have a light snack of complex carbohydrates, such as a whole-wheat sandwich, an hour before exercising to give you enough energy for your workout. If you feel faint or dizzy, or experience a severe headache, visual disturbance, heart palpitations, or any loss of fluid from the vagina, or pain in the abdomen, stop immediately and seek medical advice.

Vital Statistics

Your baby is about 5¼ to 6 inches (13 to 15 cm) from crown to rump and weighs approximately 7 ounces (200 g).

20th Week of Pregnancy

Your bump is probably quite noticeable now and it is likely to have started affecting your sense of gravity and your posture. The weight of your baby pushes your pelvis forward so that you have a natural tendency to lean back slightly, which puts a strain on your back.

Pulling in your abdominals and lengthening your back will help to correct bad posture and prevent backache. If you're finding it hard to get comfortable in bed, try putting pillows between your knees and under your bump.

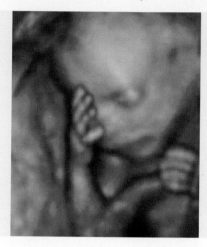

Nerve cells that serve each of your baby senses – sight, taste, smell, hearing, and touch are developing in particular areas of your baby's brain.

POSITIVE THINKING

Although you are happy to be pregnant and are excited about the new life growing inside you it's also quite natural to experience occasional pregnancy "blues." Concern about your baby, how you'll cope with labor and birth, and perhaps even how you'll be as a parent can all crowd in and make you feel dispirited at times.

Learning to relax and think positively about your pregnancy will help you overcome these feelings. Try to concentrate on all the positive aspects of being pregnant. Think about your new curvy figure, rather than the weight you've put on and keep in mind that pregnancy is a very special time.

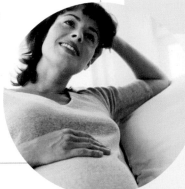

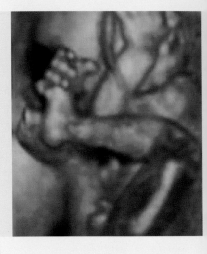

Pale pink nipples are beginning to appear over the mammary glands on your baby's chest. If your baby is a girl, her vagina, uterus, and fallopian tubes are in place. If your baby is a boy, his genitals are distinct and recognizable.

MEDITATION

Focusing on a single word or phrase can help you to achieve a profound state of relaxation. Simple, meaningless or inspiring words, short phrases or sounds work best as a mantra. If you haven't meditated before, you may find it helpful to attend a class, although it's quite possible to teach yourself through books and tapes. Meditation needs to be practiced regularly, in a comfortable environment, so make time for it each day – perhaps first thing in the morning and at night. The benefits you get from meditation will help you through pregnancy and can be taken on into parenthood.

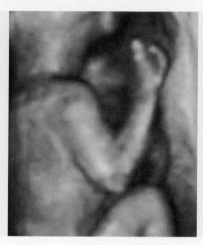

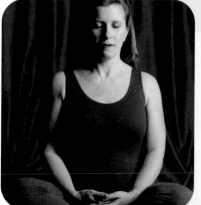

Your baby's skin is becoming thicker; there are now four layers. More vernix is accummulating.

PREGNANCY AFFIRMATIONS

Repeating a positive statement can help calm your emotions and make you cope better with discomfort. An affirmation needs to be powerful and should focus on what you want to achieve – a healthy pregnancy and baby. You may find repeating one of the following phrases helpful when in a relaxed state of mind or they may inspire you to create a more personal one of your own.

- I am (we are) happy and well.
- I am the carrier of a healthy growing baby.
- My baby is safe and well within me.
- My body is a safe haven for my baby.
- I am proud of my body. It is beautiful to the eyes and sensual to the touch.
- I can move with wonderful ease and freedom.

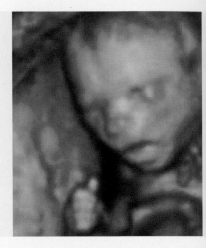

As well as the increase in neurons in his brain, there is also an increase in the complex connections required for the development of memory and thinking.

KEEPING IN TOUCH WITH YOUR BABY

You can start bonding with your baby long before the birth. By around 16 weeks, your baby can hear your heartbeat and the sound of your voice. This week, you can hear her heartbeat with a stethoscope. At 24 weeks, your baby can hear more distant sounds like your partner's voice and music. Chemicals released into your bloodstream when you laugh or are excited, or feel anger and stress cross the placenta so your baby has some experience of these feelings, too. Talking to your baby and stroking your abdomen now will help make her new world more familiar once she is born.

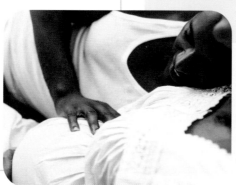

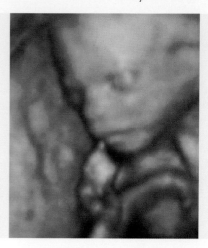

Your baby already possesses a firm handgrip. This is one of the evolutionary reflexes, which date from our earliest ancestors.

BREATHING TECHNIQUES

Breathing correctly will allow you to function better and help to relieve stress. Sit down and put your hands on your abdomen, then breathe in. You should feel your abdomen expanding as you draw air into your lungs, and then flatten again as you breathe out. For you to breathe well your shoulders need to be relaxed, so let your arms hang down and roll your shoulders backward and forward slowly to remove any tension. It's worth doing this whenever you feel tense as it will help you to relax and breathe better.

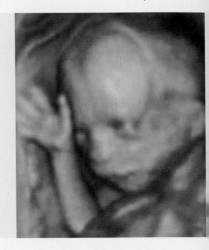

Most bones in your baby's body have hardened. When he's born, your baby will have 300 bones to your 206 because some of his bones will have to fuse together.

RELAXING BATHS

Lying in a warm – but not hot – bath will help restore your energy, while soothing away the tensions of the day. Bathing softens and cleanses your skin and relaxes your muscles, making you feel refreshed. It also provides an opportunity to practice some deep relaxation and gives you an ideal opportunity to bond with your baby.

At night, placing candles round the bath and adding a few drops of diluted essential oils such as lavender or geranium will make bathtime a wonderfully relaxing experience which will help you sleep more easily.

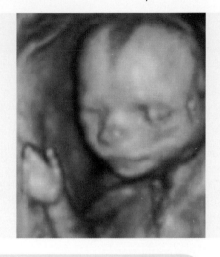

Vital Statistics

Your baby measures about 5½ to 6½ inches (14 to 16 cm) from crown to rump and weighs approximately 9 ounces (255 g).

21st Week of Pregnancy

At the end of this week, you will be half way through your pregnancy. You will need to start thinking about the type of childbirthing classes you want to attend. Although many of these don't start until the eighth month, they need to be booked in advance.

You may start to feel aches around your abdomen. This is because the ligaments on either side of the uterus stretch as your baby grows. You will be able to feel the top of your uterus in your abdomen now, just below the navel.

Your expanding uterus will have started to put pressure on your lungs, and you are likely to experience some breathlessness; if this becomes severe you should tell your healthcare provider right away.

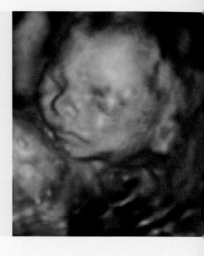

This week, tastebuds form on your baby's tongue and his sense of touch improves due to the continuing development of his brain and nerve endings.

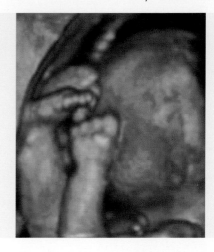

CORPSE POSITION

Before you get too large, one of the best positions in which to relax is the "corpse position" – in fact, you may find it so relaxing that you fall asleep. Before you get into the position, place a mattress, folded blanket, or some pillows on the floor and then lie down on your back. Close your eyes, and allow the tension to flow out of you by emptying your mind and allowing your limbs to flop gently.

As you get larger, change positions by lying on your side, supporting your bump and head with cushions. Take care to always go onto all fours before getting up.

While there is still plenty of space in the uterus, your baby enjoys making large movements with his legs and arms.

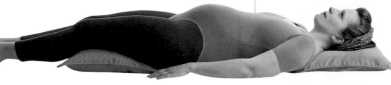

20 WEEK SCAN

You will be offered a scan between the 19th and 21st week of pregnancy to check that your baby is developing normally and that she doesn't have any major anomalies. This scan won't detect everything, but it may show any problems in the baby's major organs – most often it shows that the baby is developing well. Take your partner with you because this is a lovely chance for you both to "meet" your baby.

Depending on your hospital's policy you may be offered the opportunity to learn your baby's sex during the scan. This is something that you both need to agree on – it's much too big a secret for one of you to keep for the next 20 weeks.

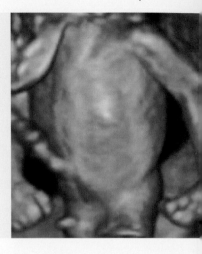

Your baby's blood is filtered by his kidneys, and the fluid he excretes passes back into the amniotic sac.

AMAZING SHAKE

This nutritious milkshake is a lovely, comforting drink for a quick pick-me-up. Use organic ingredients, if possible.

½ cup apple-strawberry juice
2 oz vanilla soy milk
½ cup oat milk
½ tablespoon rice syrup
6 ounces halved and rinsed strawberries

Place all ingredients in a blender and blend for 2-3 minutes to create a smooth, creamy drink. Serve slightly chilled in a tall glass.

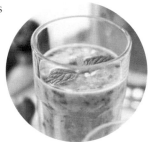

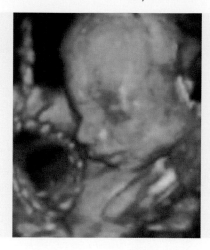

Babies at this age can make an extraordinary range of gestures. Here's a good view of the umbilical cord, which has a knotted appearance.

SELF-MASSAGE

Ease away the stresses and strains of the day by giving yourself a massage. Choose a warm, comfortable place to sit, and turn the lights down to create a peaceful atmosphere.

Begin by tapping your fingers over your scalp from front to back for two or three minutes. Then make a loose fist with one hand and pummel over your opposite shoulder; change hands. Using a small amount of oil, sweep your hand down your arms from shoulder to fingertip, and repeat several times before switching to the other arm. Finish off by kneading the side of your neck, across your shoulder, and down your upper arm, and then repeat on the other side.

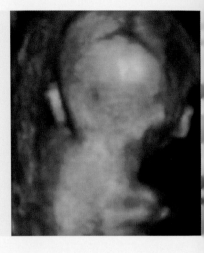

Your baby's skull consists of plates, which are not fused together so the brain is able to grow. The boneless patches that loosely join the plates won't fuse until your baby is about two years old. During birth, the bones of your baby's skull may have to overlap to enable him to pass down the birth canal.

PREVENTING VARICOSE VEINS

Swollen veins commonly appear just under the surface of the skin on your legs. You are more likely to get them if they run in the family, you're overweight, or if you stand or sit for long periods during the day.

You can help prevent them by taking regular breaks from standing and putting your feet up. Sit with your legs elevated whenever you can. If you have to sit for long periods, keep moving your legs to stimulate the circulation and flex your feet up and down. Wear support pantyhose, or ask your healthcare provider about prescription elastic stockings. Avoid tights or socks with tight tops that grip your leg, restricting the blood flow.

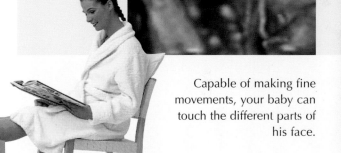

Capable of making fine movements, your baby can touch the different parts of his face.

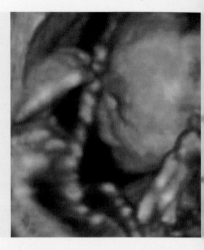

RELIEVING CRAMP

Often worse at night, leg cramps are likely to get more frequent and painful as your pregnancy progresses. No one is sure why these cramps occur – one theory links them to low levels of magnesium or calcium. Fatigue and a buildup of fluid in the legs at the end of the day are also thought to be contributing factors.

You can ease the cramp by walking about in bare feet, or by stretching and extending your legs and feet. Sometimes, vigorous leg massage will help reduce the cramp.

Vital Statistics

Your baby is about 7¼ inches (18 cm) from crown to rump and weighs approximately 10½ ounces (300 g).

22nd Week of Pregnancy

You are likely to be feeling at your sexiest now as the estrogen in your body boosts blood flow to your breasts and the pelvic area, making sexual arousal faster and more frequent than before. Some women experience their first orgasms during pregnancy. It's usually perfectly safe to make love during pregnancy, and you may enjoy it more than you ever have before.

Your weight gain is likely to be more noticeable now and you may experience an increase in appetite. Try to avoid filling up on foods such as cakes and cookies, which contain empty calories, instead eat more whole-wheat bread, rice, and pasta.

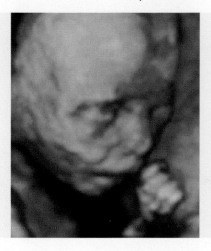

Your baby begins to have alternating periods of sleep and wakefulness. He may react to loud noises or to music. If he's sleeping, a tap on your abdomen may awaken him.

CHANGES TO MUSCLES AND JOINTS

During pregnancy the hormone relaxin softens the connective tissues around your joints, making them more flexible in preparation for the birth. This increased flexibility, however, makes your joints more susceptible to injury, so it is important to stretch your muscles gently before and after exercise, taking care not to over stretch them. You should avoid bouncy movements that put extra strain on your joints and exercises that jar your joints such as high-impact aerobics and jogging.

If your joints suffer pain as a result of this softening process you should consult your healthcare provider.

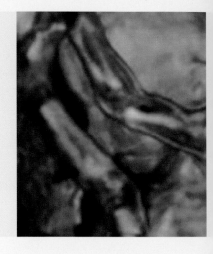

If your baby is a boy, primitive sperm have already formed in his testes.

SACROILIAC PAIN

This pain is felt in the buttocks, lower back, and hip joint – in severe cases it may even run down the leg. It is caused by increased movement in the sacroiliac joints due to hormonal softening of the ligaments. The sacroiliac joints lie between the sacrum and iliac bones at the back of the pelvis.

Sacroiliac pain can be debilitating. If you suffer from it, you should seek advice from your healthcare provider who may refer you to a cranial osteopath.

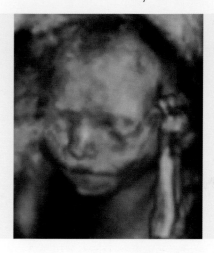

Your baby's brain starts to grow very quickly now, especially the germinal matrix, a structure in the center of his brain, which produces brain cells.

PUBIC PAIN

In later pregnancy, the pubic joint expands in preparation for birth. You may experience pain in the pubic area, which becomes noticeably worse after walking or standing, or when you're tired. Pubic pain can also be a symptom of a condition called symphysis pubis dysfunction (SPD), which can become really crippling and may persist after the birth.

You will need to see an osteopath or physiotherapist if you suffer from pubic pain, and avoid exercises which stretch the pubic joint, such as squatting or swimming breaststroke.

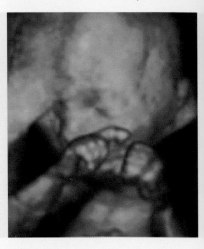

Your baby's organs are becoming specialized for particular functions although they may have different functions prior to birth. For example, your baby's liver produces more bilirubin to break down blood cells than it will once he's born.

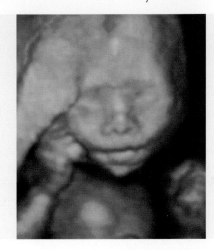

STANDING UP

You need to take care when getting up from a sitting or lying position as this can put a strain on your joints and muscles. To get yourself up, turn over so that you are on all fours, then walk your hands in and slowly bring yourself into an upright kneeling position, tilting your pelvis as you straighten up. Then lift one knee and place the foot flat on the floor. Putting both hands on your thigh, and, using your legs to lift you, push yourself up into a standing position.

Sweat glands are developing and your baby's fingernails are fully formed. They will continue to grow throughout the rest of your pregnancy.

MATERNITY LEAVE

This is the period of time you are away from work before your baby is born and after the birth. Check with your employer about your entitlement to paid and unpaid leave and other benefits. The Family and Medical Leave Act of 1993 provides that all public agencies and private-sector companies employing at least 50 workers (and with other provisos) must allow pregnant workers 12 weeks of unpaid leave.

Once you have decided when you want your leave to begin, you should write to your employer giving at least 30 days' notice of your leaving date. If you're expecting twins, you'll want to plan for more time off.

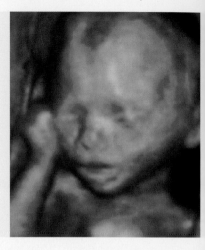

Your baby's skin is still red, although less transparent, and wrinkled. Lanugo hair covers his entire body.

HAIRCARE TIPS

Your hair will be affected by pregnancy – either becoming thicker and glossier, or thinner, greasier, or dryer than usual. Whatever changes there are to your hair, it's important to treat hair gently.

Use special shampoos and conditioners that have been specially formulated for your hair type. Don't overbrush as this will stimulate the oil glands in the scalp, which will make greasy hair greasier, and will cause dry hair to split. Avoid color treatments as pregnancy hormones can make your hair react unpredictably. It's also best to avoid treatments containing strong chemicals, such as hair relaxers and permanents, as there is a slight risk the chemicals could enter your bloodstream and affect the baby.

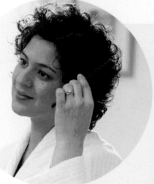

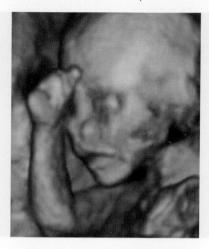

Vital Statistics

Your baby is about 7½ inches (19 cm) from crown to rump and weighs approximately 12¼ ounces (350 g).

23rd Week of Pregnancy

Your breasts have been preparing themselves for feeding your baby and they may now start leaking small amounts of colostrum, your baby's first food. If this becomes a nuisance, use breast pads or place clean, folded hankies inside your bra to absorb any leakage. If your nipples start to feel sore, try exposing your breasts to the air for a short period each day.

It's important to eat plenty of iron-rich foods now as this is when you may begin to suffer from anemia. If your healthcare provider finds that you are very anemic, you may be given iron supplements to build up your iron stores.

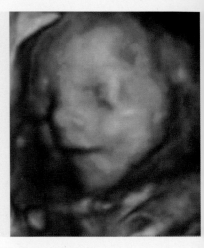

Although your baby is putting on more fat, he has a red and wrinkled appearance. This is because he produces skin at a higher rate than the fat. This skin will hang loosely. Pigmentation has begun, which accounts for the redness of your baby's skin.

CHOOSING A NAME

You and your partner may have very different views on what you'd like your baby to be called, so it's important to start discussing your ideas now. Some of the things you should consider are how the name sounds with your surname; what the name means; can it be shortened to a nickname which could be embarrassing for your child when he or she is older; or will the initials spell something unfortunate?

Write your favorites on a list and pin them up so that you can look at them often and get a feel for them. You may find it better to keep your choice to yourselves, as sometimes input from family and friends will confuse rather than help.

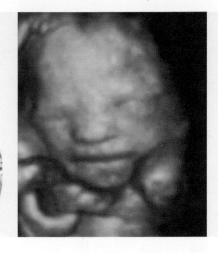

Your baby swallows small amounts of amniotic fluid, which provides him with important liquids and sugars. Swallowing this fluid can give him hiccups, which you might be able to feel.

GIRLS' NAMES

Here are some of the most popular girls' names and their meanings.

1 Emily (hard working)
2 Emma (universal strength)
3 Madison (child of Maud)
4 Hannah (full of grace)
5 Olivia (symbol of peace)
6 Abigail (father's joy)
7 Alexis (helper of mankind)
8 Ashley (from the ash tree)
9 Elizabeth (God's oath)
10 Samantha (listener)
11 Isabella (consecrated to God)
12 Sarah (princess)
13 Grace (blessing from God)
14 Alyssa (of good cheer)
15 Lauren (the laurel)

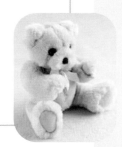

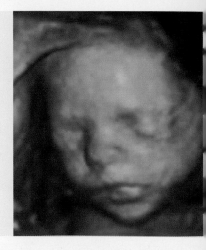

Your baby's lips have become distinct and there are tooth buds beneath his gum line. His eyes have formed, but his irises still lack pigment.

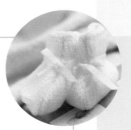

BOYS' NAMES

Here are some of the most popular boys' names and their meanings.

1 Jacob (the supplanter)
2 Michael (like the Lord)
3 Joshua (God's salvation)
4 Matthew (gift of God)
5 Andrew (manly)
6 Joseph (God multiples)
7 Ethan (steadfast and firm)
8 Daniel (God judges)
9 Chistopher (Christ bearer)
10 Anthony (priceless)
11 William (determined guardian)
12 Ryan (small king)
13 Nicholas (people triumph)
14 David (beloved one)
15 Tyler (maker of tiles or bricks)

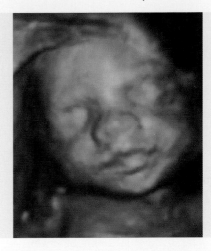

Your baby's hearing is more acute now because the bones of his inner ear have hardened. He can hear deeper voices more easily than higher-pitched ones.

DREAMS

You may experience vivid dreams that wake you during the night, leaving you feeling sad and worried. These could be caused by hormonal changes, or they may be a way of expressing anxieties that you have deep down but keep suppressed during your waking hours. Frequently, dreams at this stage of pregnancy feature the birth; you may dream that your baby is damaged or deformed in some way, or even that your pregnancy isn't real so you give birth to nothing.

Although disturbing, this type of dream is normal. You can help yourself by spending time during the day imagining your baby so that she becomes "more real." Think about what she looks likes and how she will feel.

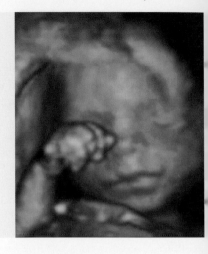

Internally, your baby's pancreas is continuing to develop; this will supply insulin, an important hormone for laying down fat in his tissues.

LIE OF YOUR BABY

Until around 32 weeks your baby has room to move around and can change position whenever she likes. After this, as she takes up more and more space in the uterus, her movements become more limited and she will eventually settle into a position that she finds comfortable, ready for birth. Most babies settle in the vertex or cephalic position, which means that their heads are down; but occasionally a baby has her feet or bottom down, a position known as breech, or, rarely, lying across the uterus in a transverse or oblique lie.

Your healthcare provider will palpate – gently press – your abdomen at your prenatal checks to feel how your baby is lying and will discuss what can be done if your baby is found to be in the wrong position for birth.

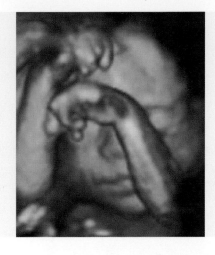

Your baby is capable of making more vigorous movements now – punching and kicking.

BIRTH PARTNER

Your birth partner has an important role to play in helping you through labor and birth. Studies have shown that women who are attended by a birth partner during labor need fewer analgesics and experience fewer medical interventions. After the birth they feel better about themselves, their labors, and their babies.

You may want your partner to be with you, or you may feel happier having your mom, sister, or a friend supporting you. Whoever you choose, it's important that you feel completely relaxed and comfortable with the person. As your birth partner will need to know what's involved, he or she should ideally have been to childbirth classes with you.

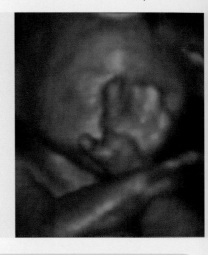

Vital Statistics

Your baby measures about 8 inches (20 cm) from crown to rump and weighs approximately 1 pound (455 g).

24th Week of Pregnancy

Your body starts to prepare for the birth by producing "practice" contractions of the uterus. Known as Braxton Hicks, after the doctor who first described them, these contractions are irregular and painless. Some women don't notice them until later in pregnancy. As your pregnancy progresses, they will become stronger, and you may be able to feel your uterus tightening if you rest your hand on your bump.

You may start to experience indigestion and heartburn as your growing abdomen puts pressure on your digestive system. Eating smaller, more frequent meals and taking a walk after you've eaten will help digestion problems.

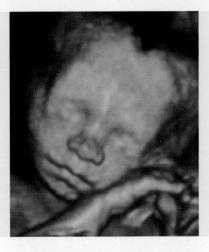

At the end of this week, with expert care, it may be possible for your baby to survive outside the uterus. However, most of his organs are still very immature, particularly his lungs.

TRAVEL SAFELY

The second trimester is a good time to take a vacation. You won't be too big yet, you'll probably be feeling pretty good and it's still safe to fly if you want to go further afield. But there are things you'll need to consider before you book a holiday.

Avoid destinations where you'll need vaccinations – although some are safe after the first 12 weeks, live vaccines like polio are not. Avoid mosquito repellents containing DEET, instead use natural alternatives such as citronella oil.

Always carry your medical notes with you in case of an emergency, so that the healthcare professionals treating you have all the information they'll need about your pregnancy.

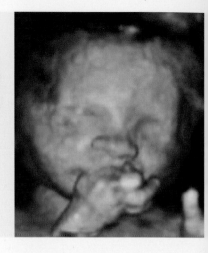

Your baby's face is filling out, and his eyes are close together on the front of his face. His eyelashes and eyebrows are well formed. His features look almost exactly as they will at birth.

FLYING

Before you book any trip, check with the airline that it's still safe for you to fly; many airlines require a letter from your doctor confirming that you are fit to fly. If you have a health problem, you'll need your healthcare provider's okay that he or she approves of your travel plans.

You are at a small, but significantly increased risk of developing deep vein thrombosis (DVT). Keep well hydrated, wear flight socks, and get up and walk around every hour to boost your circulation. When you're sitting, practice clenching your calf muscles by flexing your feet up and down 10 times every hour.

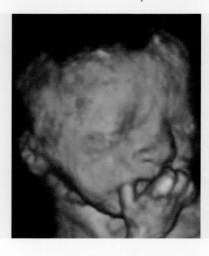

The skin on your baby's hands and feet is thicker than on the rest of his body.

TRAVELING BY CAR

Car travel poses no particular risk during pregnancy, apart from the discomfort of having to sit for along periods. Make sure you have frequent stops and get out and walk around.

When you are sitting in a car, flex your calf muscles to boost your circulation. It's important – and a legal requirement – to wear a seat belt. Position the lap part of the belt so that it sits below your bump, not above it, and keep the shoulder strap in it's normal position.

In the last weeks of pregnancy, because you'll find sitting in the same position for any length of time uncomfortable, you may want to keep any car rides to no more than half an hour.

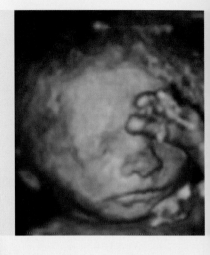

Airway passages form tubes in your baby's lungs and blood vessels, and air sacs are starting to developing in his lungs.

TAKE CARE IN THE SUN

You are more prone to dehydration during pregnancy because of your increased blood volume, so make sure you drink lots of water all through the day.

The heat will make your ankles swell, so keep your feet up as much as possible.

Protect any exposed skin with a sunscreen of factor 15 or above, and wear a long-sleeved T-shirt and a wide-brimmed hat. The sun is at its hottest between 12pm and 3pm so try to avoid being out in it during these hours.

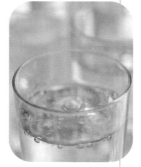

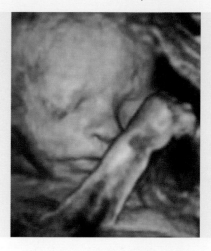

Because your baby now fills up more of the uterus, his movements are becoming restricted. Instead of cartwheeling up and down, he spends time exploring the confines of the surrounding walls.

WATCH WHAT YOU EAT

Although one of the pleasures of going on vacation is eating the local food, you need to take extra care while pregnant. Only eat in restaurants that look really clean, and don't eat food bought from stalls or markets, which might not be cooked thoroughly. Peel fruit and avoid salads unless you know for sure they've been washed properly.

Only drink the water if you know it's safe; if you're unsure, stick to still, bottled water – even when cleaning your teeth – and avoid ice in drinks. If you have an attack of diarrhea, drink plenty of water to prevent dehydration – if the diarrhea is serious seek medical advice.

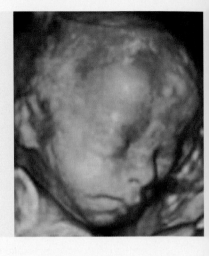

Your baby can hear very well – including your voice and stomach rumblings as well as music. He particularly likes listening to classical music.

SWIMMING

This is a great form of exercise because it gives you an all-over workout in a weightless environment without much risk of injury. The water supports your joints and ligaments as you exercise and also prevents you from becoming overheated.

Swimming will improve your circulation, increase muscle tone and strength, and build endurance. If you haven't been swimming or exercising regularly, start off slowly, and make sure you stretch well before and after your swim.

The water temperature should be comfortable – don't swim in water that's too cold or too hot.

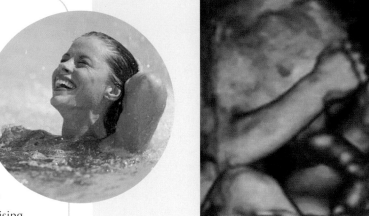

Vital Statistics

Your baby now measures about 8½ inches (21 cm) from crown to rump and weighs approximately 1¼ pounds (540 g).

25th Week of Pregnancy

Your pregnancy is well advanced and you may be finding that your increased weight is starting to take its toll, making everything seem more of an effort. Try to plan your life to make things easier for yourself.

Cook batches of meals on the weekend and freeze them ready to eat at night when you are feeling at your most exhausted. Take time out – sit with your feet up, read a book or watch TV rather than rushing to do jobs around the house. Your next prenatal appointment will be due soon, so think about any questions or concerns you may have so that you can discuss them with your healthcare provider.

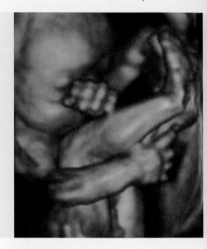

By now your baby has settled into a daily pattern of sleep and activity. His kicks and prods tell you when he is most active.

BREASTFEEDING

Your breasts have been preparing themselves to produce milk since the beginning of your pregnancy. After the birth, they will produce colostrum – a high-protein liquid rich in antibodies, which protect your baby from infection and help to build a strong immune system. After a few days, colostrum changes to breast milk, which contains all the nutrients your baby needs, in the right quantities, for the first six months of her life.

Breastfeeding has many benefits for you, too. As well as helping your body to recover more quickly after the birth, breastfeeding for at least six months significantly reduces the risk of pre-menopausal breast cancer and can protect against osteoporosis and ovarian cancer.

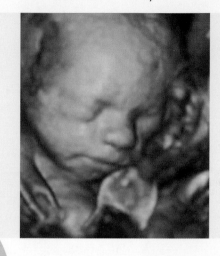

Your baby's nostrils begin to open. High inside your baby's gums, his permanent teeth are developing in buds. They won't descend until his baby teeth start to fall out when he's around six years old.

BREAST CARE

As your breasts prepare themselves for breastfeeding, the glands that look like little bumps on the areola – the dark area surrounding the nipples – produce natural lubricants to soften the nipples. It's best to wash your breasts with plain water, as using bath products containing soap will remove these natural oils. Gently massage your breasts after bathing and use whatever moisturizer you are using for your abdomen on your breasts, but avoid the nipple area. In the last month you can begin to use a tiny amount of pure lanolin or nipple care cream, which is especially made for breastfeeding. Expose your breasts to the air or mild sunshine occasionally, and spend some time without a bra around the house or in bed at night.

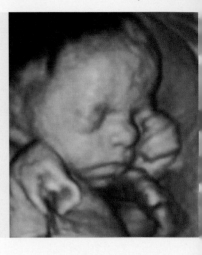

Most of his vital organs are well developed except for his lungs. Blood vessels continue to develop there.

BOTTLE FEEDING

If for any reason you can't, or you choose not to breastfeed, you will need to feed your baby with an infant formula. These are usually based on cow's milk. Although formula milk doesn't give your baby the same protection as breast milk, it does contain all the vitamins and minerals your baby needs to thrive for the first six months. You will need to buy bottles and nipples, a bottle brush, and sterilizing equipment. Good hygiene is very important when you bottle feed.

If for medical reasons your baby is unable to digest cow's milk your healthcare provider will be able to suggest an alternative infant formula.

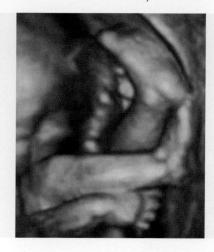

Your baby is quite dexterous. The nerves around his mouth and lips are more sensitive and he enjoys sucking body parts, such as his knees.

ABDOMINAL MASSAGE

Massaging your bump with a moisturizing cream or oil is relaxing and a lovely way for you or your partner to communicate with your baby. Make sure the room is warm and get comfortable before you start. Put the answering machine on so that you won't be disturbed and turn the lights down, or close the curtains. You may find it helpful to play soothing music, or you may simply prefer to lie quietly and sing or talk to your baby as you gently stroke your abdomen. Your baby's movements are likely to respond to the touch of your hand so you'll have a real feeling of communication.

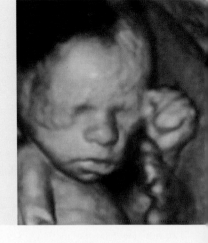

The umbilical cord is thick and resilient and continues to be your baby's lifeline, delivering oxygen and nutrients from your circulation via the placenta. Ever present, it may be a source of consolation to your baby.

ITCHING

It's quite normal to experience some itching, especially around your bump where the skin has stretched.

If your palms and soles of your feet become red and itchy, this could be a harmless condition known as palmar erythema, which is caused by an increase in estrogen. However, if you develop severe itching on your hands and feet during the last three months, this may be a sign of pregnancy cholestasis, a rare but potentially dangerous liver disorder. Other symptoms of cholestasis may include dark urine and pale stools and jaundice.

Any severe itching should be reported to your healthcare provider and if cholestasis is suspected your condition will need to be carefully monitored.

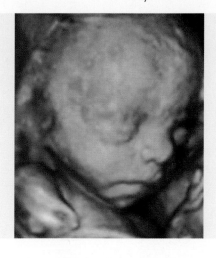

Although still thin-skinned and skinny, your baby has become better proportioned.

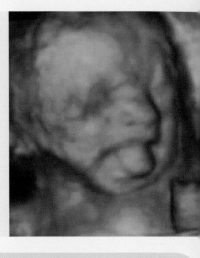

EYE CHANGES

Like your other organs, your eyes are also affected by pregnancy hormones, and you may notice some changes in your vision. If you wear glasses or contact lenses, fluid retention, especially during the last trimester, can make your current prescription either too weak or too strong. However, you don't need to get your eyes re-tested as this will right itself in the weeks after the birth.

If you wear contact lenses, you may find that they become uncomfortable and irritate your eyes. This is because the fluid pressure inside your eyes decreases slightly during pregnancy, causing your eyes to change shape.

Vital Statistics
Your baby is about 8¾ inches (22 cm) from crown to rump and weighs approximately 1½ pounds (700 g).

26th Week of Pregnancy

Congratulations! You're now in your last trimester of pregnancy and you can look forward to more rapid weight gain. Your uterus is the size of a soccer ball and is pushing up against your diaphragm and ribs, and you may find that you quickly become out of breath. Try sitting or standing as tall as you can and concentrate on taking slow, deep breaths until the feeling of breathlessness has passed.

The uterus is also putting pressure on your stomach so that indigestion and heartburn can become a problem, especially if you've eaten a big meal late at night. If heartburn prevents you from eating properly, or getting to sleep at night, ask your healthcare provider about antacids that are suitable to take during pregnancy.

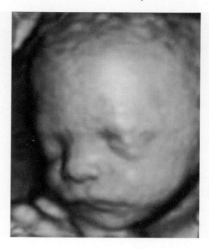

Your baby's vital organs are all well developed except for his lungs. Though the lungs' network of blood vessels is increasing, the lungs still need many weeks' growth to mature sufficiently.

HEARTBURN

This is an unpleasant burning sensation which you feel in the upper part of your abdomen near your breastbone. It's caused by the valve at the top of the stomach relaxing and allowing acid to pass back into the esophagus. Having small, frequent meals and avoiding spicy, fatty, and greasy foods will help to prevent this from happening.

As soon as you start to experience heartburn, try eating dry crackers or drinking a glass of milk; these will help to neutralize the acid. As heartburn most commonly occurs at night, not eating too late and lying propped up in bed may also be beneficial.

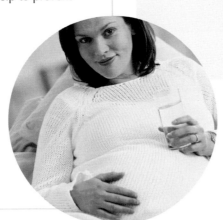

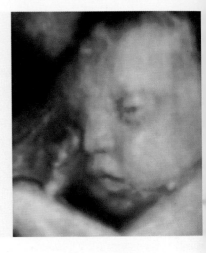

The long development of your baby's eyes is now complete as the final layers of his retina in the backs of his eyes have formed. He can now open his eyelids some of the time.

PELVIC TILT

The extra weight you are carrying pulls your center of gravity forward so that your back arches, causing you to lean back slightly. This unnatural position can lead to aches and pains in the small of your back. Practicing the pelvic tilt regularly will strengthen the muscles in this area and help to prevent backache.

Kneel on all fours with your back straight. Tilt your pelvis by clenching your buttock muscles and arching your back. Hold for a few seconds, then release. Alternatively, stand up straight and lengthen your spine by pulling your tailbone down and lifting the front of your pelvis upward. Do this whenever you are standing so that it becomes part of your normal posture.

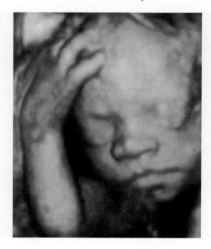

Your baby has all his fingernails as well as eyebrows and eyelashes. He occasionally makes breathing movements although there is no air in his lungs. The movements, however, help his lungs to mature.

PETS

You are not likely to be in any danger from family pets during pregnancy, providing that you take a little extra care. Although a dog, even a large one, doesn't pose a risk in itself, it could unintentionally hurt you by jumping up and causing you to lose your balance. It makes sense, if you have a dog, to keep it under control both in the home and outside; after all, he'll need to be well-behaved once your baby arrives.

Cats are more of a risk as they may carry a rare infection called toxoplasmosis. This infection is present in cat feces so, as far as possible, have someone else change your cat's litter box. If this isn't possible, wear gloves and wash your hands afterward. Cats who are confined indoors all the time pose no risk.

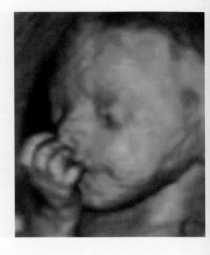

Brain scans show that your baby does respond to touch and sound. His pulse may quicken, he may move his arms or legs, or he may even move in rhythm to music.

TOXOPLASMOSIS

This rare infection can be caught through contact with an outdoor cat's feces, and by eating unwashed vegetables or under-cooked meat. If you become infected, there is a chance that the infection could be passed on to your baby. If this happens early in pregnancy, the effect on your baby's development will be greater than if the infection is passed on later in pregnancy.

Some doctors automatically screen for toxoplasmosis, others don't unless your circumstances put you at risk. If toxoplasmosis is suspected, you will be given a blood test. If these confirm toxoplasmosis, you will be referred to a specialist who will be able to advise you on the possible implications of the infection.

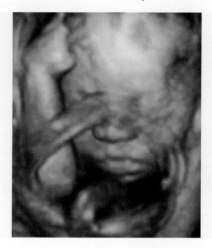

Your baby will soon start to put on weight in the form of fat cells. Until now, most of the increase in his weight has been due to the accumulation of protein, which was needed to build up his cells.

BABY'S MOVEMENTS

Your baby starts to move as early as the seventh or eighth week of pregnancy, although you won't become aware of these movements until around the 18th week, or even as late as 24 weeks. For you to feel your baby's movements, she needs to be big enough to make her presence felt through nudging and poking your insides. What you can feel is your baby pushing the uterus against muscles and organs such as your abdominal wall. As your baby gets bigger, she has less space to move around in and her movements become more pronounced. You will be able to feel quite strong kicks against your bladder or ribs.

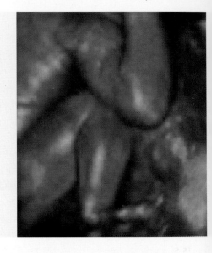

Your baby's spine is getting stronger and more supple to support his growing body.

ROUND LIGAMENT PAIN

You may experience a pain on one or both sides of your abdomen, or near your groin, the severity of which can vary from a dull ache to a sharp stabbing pain that may get stronger when you move about and fade if you lie down. Known as round ligament pain, this occurs as the enlarging uterus stretches the ligaments that run down either side of it and attach the top of the uterus to the labia.

Although uncomfortable, the pain will usually have gone, or at least have decreased considerably by the end of this week. You can help yourself by resting with your feet up as much as possible.

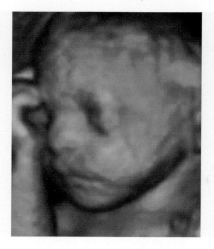

Vital Statistics
Your baby measures just over 9 inches (23 cm) from crown to rump and weighs approximately 2 pounds (910 g).

27th Week of Pregnancy

If measured, your cholesterol levels would appear to be quite high. Cholesterol is a vital building block for the pregnancy hormones manufactured by the placenta. The most important of which, progesterone, is essential for breast development and to relax the uterine muscles.

Your pelvic floor muscles are being put under pressure by your enlarged uterus, and you may find that you leak small amounts of urine when you laugh or sneeze. This is known as stress incontinence. It's important to do your pelvic floor exercises regularly to strengthen these muscles. Wearing panty-liners will stop stress incontinence becoming an embarrassment.

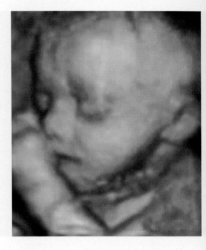

Rounder and plumper due to increased amounts of fat being deposited under his skin, your baby would have about an 80 percent chance of surviving if he was born this week.

GESTATIONAL DIABETES

This is a form of diabetes that occurs when the body can't make enough insulin to meet the extra demands of pregnancy. It is determined by a blood sugar test, which can be done at different times. Most commonly it is carried out between the 26th and 28th week. You are more at risk of the condition if you're overweight, an older mom, have a family history of type-2 diabetes, previously had a big baby, or had two or more previous pregnancies.

If you develop gestational diabetes your baby may grow exceptionally large and have to be delivered early. Sometimes diabetes can be controlled by changes to the diet, but between 10 and 30 percent of the women afflicted need insulin injections during their pregnancy. The condition disappears after the birth.

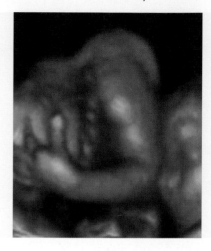

As your twins grow, space in the uterus decreases, leading to competition but also a closer companionship.

BONDING

Mother, and sometimes father, and child become attached to one another before birth. A mother's bond is physiological because she provides nutrients and the chemicals that cause upset or pleasure. Some scientists also believe that mothers communicate sympathetically with their unborn babies, through dreams, for example. The senses are heightened in pregnancy, and it is often possible for pregnant women to gain a close connection with their babies. Communicating with your baby can be done through song, music, or sounds, as well as touching your tummy frequently. Meditation may also help to increase your receptivity to your baby.

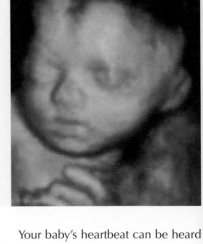

Your baby's heartbeat can be heard by anyone putting his or her ear to your abdomen.

GOING BACK TO WORK

Although it may be hard to decide at this stage of your pregnancy whether you want to go back to work or not after the birth, it is something you need to think about. You may want to leave it as long as possible before you return to your old job, or you may prefer to consider more flexible working hours, perhaps even going part-time.

It's a good idea to find out now what choices you have, and what you need to do if you want to change your work pattern. Your employer or your human resources department will be able to tell you what your options are, and how you go about negotiating any changes to your working hours.

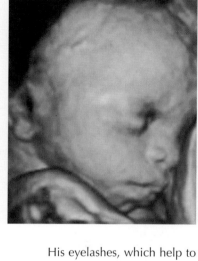

His eyelashes, which help to protect his delicate eyeballs from harmful matter, are fully grown.

CHILDCARE

If you have decided to return to work after the birth you will need to organize childcare well in advance. Many day nurseries are booked up months ahead, so you may need to get your baby's name on a waiting list now. And, if you're thinking about employing a nanny, it's a good idea to research agencies or individuals.

Alternatively, you might want to consider sharing the care with your partner, or having a relative look after your child. The most important factor is to make sure that your child has continuity of care in a safe and happy environment.

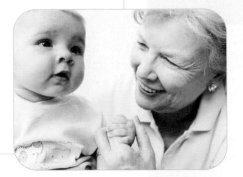

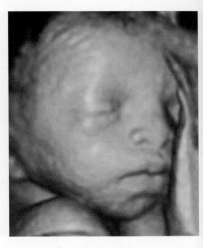

The taste buds on your baby's tongue and inside his cheeks are fully functional now. His higher brain functions are becoming more sophisticated.

FORGETFULNESS

If your short-term memory isn't as good as it used to be don't worry; many women find that they become forgetful during pregnancy. During the first trimester you are likely to be distracted by nausea, fatigue, and the hormonal changes your body is undergoing. Toward the end of pregnancy, worry about how you will cope with the enormous life changes that are ahead of you, coupled with feelings of exhaustion, can make you forgetful.

Try carrying a notebook so you can write reminders to yourself of important things you need to do, keeping a detailed diary and putting items you use often in the same place so that you can find them easily. Above all, remain calm – any forgetfulness will soon pass once your baby arrives.

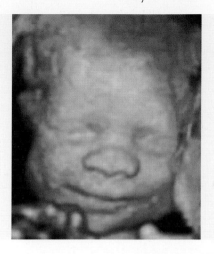

Your baby's lungs continue to grow but the air sacs lack a vital substance that keeps them inflated. He is still not able to breathe for himself.

3-D ULTRASOUNDS

Images of this new and exciting ultrasound technique are shown throughout this book. Using the same ultrasound waves as a conventional scan, the waves are collected in volumes – rather than thin slices – which can then be displayed in three dimensions. This provides a lifelike representation of the surface features of the baby. The images can be updated three or four times each second (called 4-D) so that the movements, facial expressions, and moods of the baby can be seen clearly by the parents and healthcare professionals. Although, at the moment, few couples have the opportunity to view their babies with this technique, the images give all expectant parents the opportunity to see how a baby develops and behaves in the uterus.

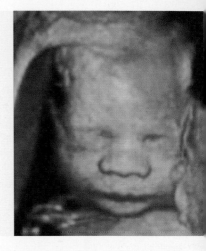

Vital Statistics

Your baby is about 9½ inches (24 cm) from crown to rump and weighs approximately 2 pounds 2 ounces (1 kg).

28th Week of Pregnancy

You'll find your relationship with your baby is getting closer as you become familiar with his movements and sleep periods. You are probably very protective of your "bump."

It is a good idea to "test" for your baby's movements. During one hour in the morning and evening, you should see whether you can feel 10 movements. If so, everything is okay. If not, you should contact your healthcare provider.

Your body may be starting to feel the effects of the enormous strain it's under, and you are likely to experience some common late-pregnancy symptoms such as constipation, cramp, breathlessness, and backache. If any of these become a problem, ask your healthcare provider for advice.

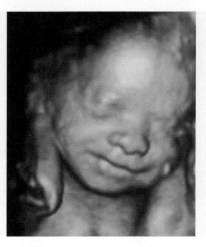

Your baby's lungs are capable of breathing air although, if born now, he would find it very difficult to breathe properly. He occasionally makes regular breathing movements.

ADDITIONAL CALORIES

You'll need to increase your calorie intake now by around 250 to 300 calories a day to meet the demands of your growing baby. This can easily be achieved by eating an extra bowl of cereal with low-fat milk, or a banana with a glass of milk. If these additional calories don't satisfy your appetite, include some other healthy snacks, such as a piece of fruit or some raw vegetables.

If you have any concerns about the amount of weight you are putting on, ask your healthcare provider to monitor your weight gain over the next few weeks.

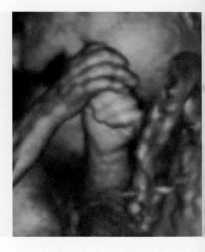

Space in the uterus is becoming restricted due to your baby's increasing weight, but this means he is becoming better acquainted with the various parts of his own body.

SWEET VEGETABLE TEA

Taken at least three times a week, this tea will give you stable, slow-release energy that creates vitality.

Put 3 cups spring water in a pan and bring to the boil on a medium heat.

Add ½ onion, finely sliced; ½ carrot, washed and finely sliced; a handful of cabbage, washed and shredded; and 1-inch slice of hard green winter squash, washed, seeds removed and finely sliced. Simmer, uncovered, for about 2 minutes.

Cover and simmer on a low heat for 15-20 minutes.

Strain the vegetables and drink the remaining liquid while still hot.

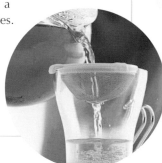

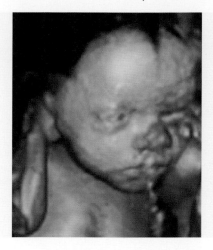

Although it is dark in the uterus, your baby can open his eyes for periods of time. His umbilical cord could be right in front of his nose, but he won't be able to see it.

HEADACHES

Tension headaches are quite common during the first trimester and may be brought on by fluctuating hormones and changes in your blood circulation. Sinus headaches, due to congestion of the mucus membranes caused by pregnancy hormones, are also common. However, headaches in the second or third trimester could be a sign of pre-eclampsia, a serious pregnancy-induced condition that needs immediate treatment (see also page 200).

If you have persistent headache, which is severe or accompanied by visual disturbances, or puffy hands and face, you should consult your healthcare provider right away.

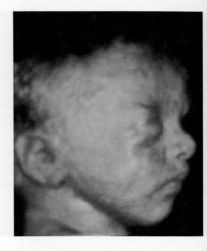

Your baby is developing scalp hair, especially on the back of his head. The network of nerves to his ear is now complete, and he can hear more and more.

EDEMA

Swelling of the feet, hands, and fingers, or edema, is common in later pregnancy. Your body swells because of a natural accumulation of fluid in the tissues. Edema is most notice-able at the end of the day, or if you have been standing for a long period and in hot weather.

To help expel the excess fluid drink plenty of water. Don't stand for long periods and avoid wearing tight clothing or shoes; sit with your feet up when you can. If your hands are swollen, hold them up above the level of your heart rather than down by your sides. Report any swelling to your healthcare provider as there is a slight chance that it could be a sign of pre-eclampsia.

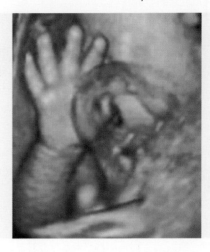

The umbilical cord is very strong and can withstand being squeezed and twisted by your baby. Babies frequently grip their cords.

PRE-ECLAMPSIA

This condition only arises during pregnancy. It is rare before 28 weeks, but can occur up to several days after the birth. You are at higher risk if you're a first-time mom, a teenage mom, are carrying more than one baby, or you've had pre-eclampsia before.

Pre-eclampsia is caused by damage to the placenta, which leads to problems with your circulation and shows up as raised blood pressure, protein in the urine, and swelling. In severe cases it may cause bad headaches, blurring or flashing lights in the vision, pain below the ribs, and vomiting. If you develop pre-eclampsia, you and your baby will be closely monitored. If the condition starts to deteriorate, your baby will need to be delivered early.

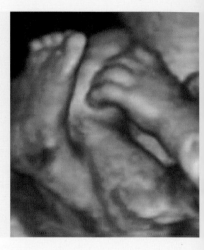

Your baby is now about one-third of his estimated birth weight. Baby fat is accumulating underneath his skin and his muscles are becoming well developed.

COUVADE SYNDROME

Very occasionally, a man can share some of the same pregnancy symptoms as his partner. He puts on weight, suffers from morning sickness and fatigue, and may even need to take more trips to the bathroom. Known as Couvade syndrome, it usually begins in the first trimester and continues until the birth, when the man experiences stomach cramps while his partner is in labor. Although nerves have been blamed, research has proved that the condition is real. Men who have undergone infertility treatment or who were adopted are more susceptible to couvade.

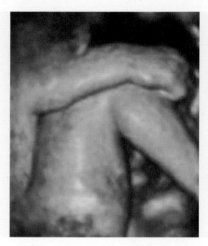

Vital Statistics

Your baby is about 10 inches (25 cm) from crown to rump and weighs approximately 2½ pounds (1.1 kg).

29th Week of Pregnancy

You will be having prenatal checks every two weeks now as your healthcare providers will want to monitor your progress closely. You will be given a blood test to check for anemia and, if you're Rhesus negative, you'll also have an antibody check.

Now is a good time to write your birth plan, outlining how you would like your labor and birth to be managed. Discuss your ideas with your partner first and then with your healthcare professionals.

Don't worry; writing a birth plan does not commit you to having a certain type of birth, you can change your mind at any time until you actually have your baby.

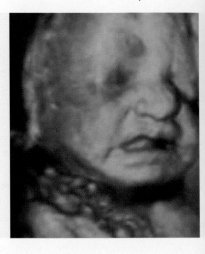

Your baby's brain is growing quite quickly now and the soft bones of his skull are expanding to accommodate it. Even if wrapped around your baby's neck, his umbilical cord is able to maintain blood flow.

ANEMIA

At this stage of pregnancy, anemia is common because your blood volume has increased by a third, and more iron is needed to make enough red blood cells to carry oxygen around your body. The main symptom of anemia is tiredness, although in severe cases you may also feel faint, dizzy, breathless, and see spots in front of your eyes. If you experience any of these symptoms, you should contact your healthcare provider immediately. Anemia is easily treatable with iron tablets, but iron-rich foods, such as red meat, kidney beans, fish, and spinach should also form a major part of your diet.

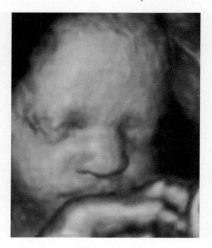

Your baby is capable of demonstrating lots of expressions; scans have revealed babies grimacing, smiling, and even laughing!

CYSTITIS

This is an infection of the bladder that requires immediate treatment with pregnancy-approved antibiotics and it could put your baby at risk. Symptoms of cystitis include wanting to pass urine frequently – but only managing a few drops – burning and stinging while passing urine, fever, and abdominal pain. Urine infections can lead to premature labor and should always be treated seriously.

To help speed recovery, drink plenty of water to flush out bacteria from your bladder. Antibiotics can interfere with the bacterial balance in your intestines, so eat plain yogurt containing active cultures to help restore "good" bacteria.

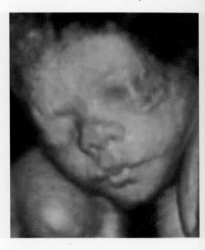

The surface of your baby's brain is becoming more and more irregular as grooves and indentations form. These are known as *gyri* and *sulci* and are a result of connections being made between nerve cells.

BIRTH PLAN

Making a plan for how you would like your labor and the delivery of your baby to be managed will help you to achieve the kind of birth you want. It is also a good way to identify any issues that you are not sure about, and will give you a chance to discuss your ideas with your healthcare providers. Some hospitals have a formal plan for you to fill in, others are happy to accept your own notes – either way, you need to take your plan with you when you give birth. It's important for your birth partner to be involved in the making of your plan so that he or she is aware of your wishes.

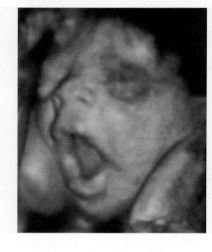

Nobody knows why babies yawn in the uterus, but they do! In fact, they begin to yawn as early as 12 weeks of pregnancy.

SHOULDER DE-TENSER

The stresses and strains of late pregnancy can make you tired and your body feel tense, especially across your shoulders. Simple shoulder rolls can help.

Stand with your feet about hip-width apart, with your knees relaxed and your arms by your sides. Tilt your pelvis and tighten your abdominals to lift your baby. Rotate your right shoulder forward, raise it toward your ear, then circle it behind you in a large movement, taking it back and down again. Do eight reps with one shoulder, then repeat on the other side.

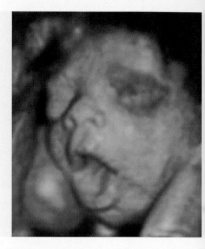

Babies spend most of the time in the uterus asleep but when awake, your baby is still able to stretch and kick you, though space is becoming limited. You should feel frequent kicks throughout the day.

RECTUS DIASTASES

This is a separation of the two halves of the rectus abdominus – the muscle that runs down the middle of your abdomen – that sometimes occurs during pregnancy. You can check for it by lying on your back with your knees bent. Place your fingertips 1 to 2 inches below your belly button, fingers pointing toward your feet. Lift your head as high as you can – if you feel a ridge protruding from the midline of your abdomen, that's diastasis. If present, you'll need to consult your healthcare provider about what you can – or cannot – do.

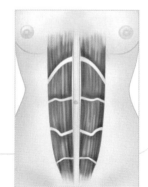

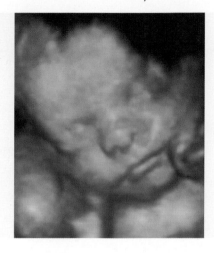

Even when babies sleep their brains are working, and during part of this time their eyes respond with little reflex movements, known as rapid eye movements or REM. In adults these are associated with dreaming, but we don't know if babies dream.

DRAWING OUT NIPPLES

Flat or retracted nipples can make breastfeeding difficult, although not impossible. To check your nipples try holding each breast between your forefinger and thumb, about ½ to 1 inch outside the areola, and applying gentle pressure. If your nipples retract into the areola or remain very flat, you may need to wear specially designed breast shells that will help them to protrude. Your healthcare provider will be able to advise you about breast shells and may suggest when you should wear them.

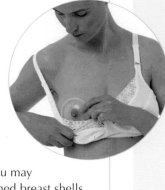

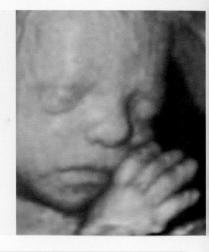

Vital Statistics

Your baby is about 10¼ inches (26 cm) from crown to rump and weighs approximately 2 pounds 12 ounces (1.25 kg).

30th Week of Pregnancy

You may find you are having to urinate more frequently as your enlarging uterus starts putting pressure on your bladder again.

Extreme tiredness may also be a problem now, especially if you are having to get up frequently in the night to visit the bathroom. A warm, milky drink before bedtime will help you sleep. Warming milk releases tryptophan, a naturally occurring amino acid that makes you sleepy. Try to get plenty of rest during the day, and go to bed early with a good book – even if you're not asleep your body will be relaxed.

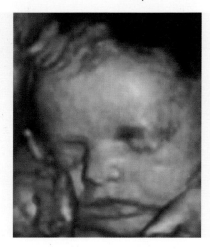

Your baby continues to put on fat and is becoming plumper and less wrinkled. If he was born now, he'd be better able to keep himself warm.

CHILDBIRTH CLASSES

These classes are designed to help you prepare for labor and birth. The teacher will talk through the birth process and give you the chance to ask questions and discuss any concerns you may have in a relaxed, informal atmosphere. Meeting in a group can be very supportive as all the women there will be going through the same experiences as you so they'll understand how you feel. Birth partners are usually encouraged to attend. Going to class will enable your partner to become more involved in your pregnancy and understand his (or her) role in the birth.

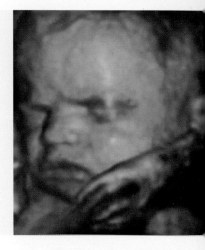

Your baby can hear well and may respond to a loud noise with a kick.

CHOOSING A CLASS

Classes are usually run by hospitals and birth centers, or by midwives at community health centers. Your healthcare provider should be able to give you details of classes available in your area. Alternatively, you can attend a private course run by a specialist childbirth teacher. These private courses are usually based on a particular philosophy, so make sure that this is in keeping with your views on childbirth. Look for classes which cater for around five to seven couples so that you get some individual attention as well as group discussion.

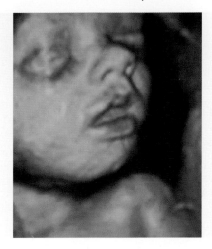

There are as many neural circuits in your baby's brain now as there will be when he is born.

LAMAZE AND BRADLEY CLASSES

These are two specialist classes that may be available to you. Teachers of Lamaze childbirth classes encourage active birth, through movement and breathing techniques. Intensive training and practice is used to teach you how to give positive responses to contractions rather than negative ones. Your birth partner trains with you so that he or she can assist you through labor and delivery.

Bradley-based classes start as soon as you are pregnant and focus on partner-coached "natural" childbirth, with a lot of emphasis on good diet and prenatal exercise. During labor, you are encouraged to use deep abdominal breathing and inner focus to cope with the contractions.

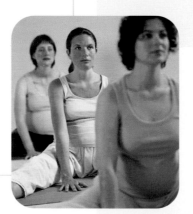

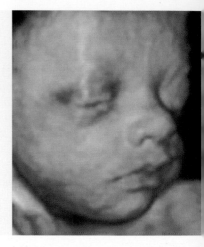

Your baby's skeleton continues to harden. His brain, muscles, and lungs continue to mature.

ELECTIVE CESAREAN

This operation is planned in advance because of some medical complication. The most common reason for an elective cesarean is a previous cesarean section. But you may be offered a cesarean if you have a medical condition such as pre-eclampsia, are carrying more than one baby, your baby is considered to be too large to fit through your pelvis, or she is lying in the wrong position in the uterus.

The operation, which is usually carried out before you actually go into labor, is generally performed using a spinal anesthetic so that you remain awake during the procedure.

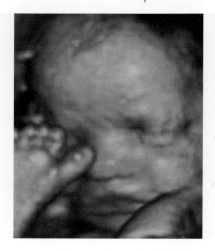

He still has some room in the uterus in which to bring his feet up to his face. Soon, he won't be able to do this.

PREPARING FOR A CESAREAN

If you know you are having a cesarean, advance planning will help to make this a more satisfying experience.

Go to childbirth classes that include information on cesarean birth; in this way you can find out as much as possible about the procedure beforehand. Make a birth plan based on this information and discuss it with your healthcare provider to see what's practical. Ask if you and your partner can look around the labor and childbirth areas so that when you have your baby the room where you give birth will be familiar.

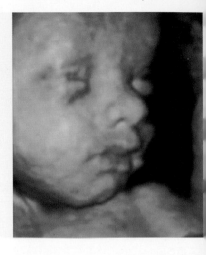

Your baby's liver is no longer responsible for the production of red blood cells; his bone marrow has completely taken over the task.

PRE-TERM LABOR

This is when contractions start before the 37th week of pregnancy. If this happens you will be monitored closely as your baby may be too immature to cope on her own if she's born too early. The reasons for pre-term labor are unclear, but bladder or uterine infections, problems with the placenta, or being pregnant with more than one baby are thought to be among the causes. Pre-term contractions should always be reported to your healthcare provider immediately. Depending on your stage of pregnancy, you may be given drugs to try to delay, slow, or stop the labor.

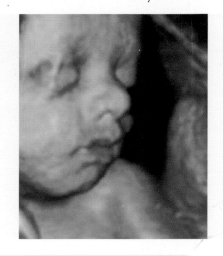

Vital Statistics

Your baby measures about 10¾ inches (27 cm) from crown to rump and weighs approximately 3 pounds (1.36 kg).

31st Week of Pregnancy

As you get larger you get slower and clumsier, and you may find that you are dropping things and tripping over your own feet. This is partly because your increased weight affects your balance, and partly because your fingers, toes, and other joints are all loosened by pregnancy hormones. You should take care when climbing stairs, walking on uneven surfaces, and when you're out in wet or icy weather.

If you do have a fall, your baby is unlikely to be hurt because she's well protected inside the uterus, but you should report any fall to your healthcare provider just to make sure everything is all right.

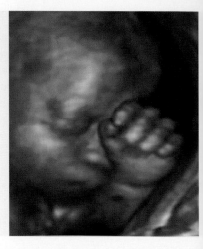

Your baby has pronounced daily rhythms of sleep and wakefulness. However, he is most likely to be active when you are trying to sleep.

CONSTIPATION

Hard and difficult-to-pass stools can be an uncomfortable side effect of pregnancy. Constipation occurs because pregnancy hormones slow down the transit of food through your digestive tract and the growing uterus puts pressure on your rectum. Prenatal iron supplements can also make constipation worse. Taking regular exercise, eating high-fiber foods such as cereals and whole-grain bread, and drinking plenty of water can help relieve the problem. Drink prune juice every day and make sure you always go to the bathroom when you feel the urge. Your healthcare provider may also suggest taking a fiber supplement.

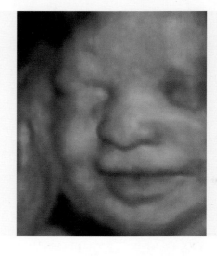

Because his cerebral cortex has matured enough to support consciousness, your baby is capable of feeling and remembering.

HEMORRHOIDS

Also known as piles, hemorrhoids are varicose veins in your back passage or anus. They are caused by pregnancy and aggravated by constipation and straining. Hemorrhoids can be itchy and painful and in severe cases may even bleed.

Apply an ice pack to relieve any discomfort and relieve itching with a soothing cream. If you experience any bleeding you should seek advice from your healthcare provider.

You can help prevent hemorrhoids – or stop them from becoming any worse – by eating high-fiber foods and drinking plenty of water so that your stools remain soft and regular. Hemorrhoids usually disappear without the need for treatment in the weeks after the birth.

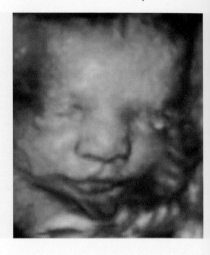

The hair on your baby's head is increasing and becoming thicker while the lanugo, or body hair, is disappearing. Whatever is left will rub off in the weeks after birth.

HIGH-FIBER FOODS

Fiber is essential for a healthy digestive system and for preventing constipation. It also helps to maintain your blood sugar levels. There are two types of fiber – soluble and insoluble. Soluble fiber is found in foods such as apples, pears, oats, rye, and legumes. It helps you feel full for longer and maintains an even release of sugars into the blood. Insoluble fiber, found in beans, fruit, green leafy vegetables, lentils, and whole-grain cereals aids the progress of food through your digestive system and helps prevent constipation. For fiber to work effectively you need to drink plenty of fluids. Try to maintain a fluid intake of at least 8 glasses a day.

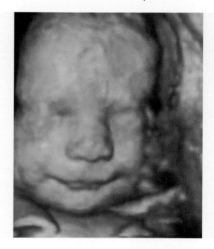

Your baby's skin is looking less wrinkled because he has put on more baby fat. He is looking a lot rounder.

BRAXTON HICKS CONTRACTIONS

Named after the doctor who first described them, these are "practice" contractions which stretch the lower part of the uterus. You will feel a tightening across your abdomen, which lasts from a few seconds to a minute and then fades away. You may find they become stronger and more pronounced toward the end of pregnancy. It's a good idea to use them to practice breathing and relaxation techniques for labor. Breathe out as your bump goes hard and take slow, deep breaths while you relax your body. As the contraction fades away, take a deep breath in.

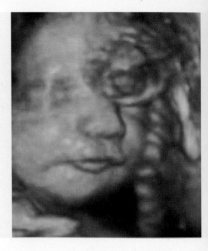

Your baby is becoming more aware; he is able to feel your uterus massaging him when you have Braxton Hicks contractions. If he hears a noise, he will react to it with a kick.

NECK RELAXER

You can release tension in your neck with this simple exercise.

Sit in a comfortable position. Tilt your pelvis and tighten your abdominal muscles. Rest your hands on your knees, press your shoulders down and lengthen your spine. Slowly tilt your head over to the left side, pressing your ear toward your shoulder – do not raise your shoulder toward your ear. Pause, then return to the upright position before repeating on the right side. Do as often as you like.

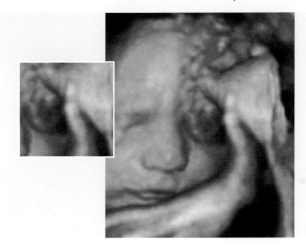

Your baby's fingernails and toenails are growing. At the same time, his skeleton is hardening more and more. If your baby is a girl, her clitoris will be relatively prominent because her labia are still small and haven't covered it yet.

CARPAL TUNNEL SYNDROME

The carpal tunnel houses the tendons and nerves that run down from the front of the wrists to the fingers. The swelling you get in your hands in pregnancy causes the carpal tunnel to swell too, putting pressure on these nerves. Known as carpal tunnel syndrome, this swelling causes pain in the wrist, and pins and needles and stiffness in the fingers and joints of the hand. The symptoms tend to be worse at night; try sleeping with your hands raised on a pillow to help prevent fluid building up. You can ease stiffness first thing in the morning by hanging your hands over the side of the bed and giving them a vigorous shake.

If you experience a lot of discomfort, your healthcare provider may suggest wearing a splint. Carpal tunnel syndrome should disappear in the days following delivery.

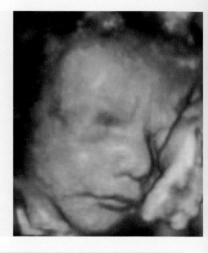

Vital Statistics

Your baby is about 11 inches (28 cm) from crown to rump and weighs approximately 3½ pounds (1.59 kg).

32nd Week of Pregnancy

You are likely to have gained around 19 pounds (8.6 kg) by this stage of your pregnancy. This extra weight is not just your baby – the placenta, amniotic fluid, enlarged breasts, and uterus, an increase in blood volume and in your body's stores of fat, protein, and fluid all contribute to these additional pounds.

This extra weight is likely to make you feel more breathless and uncomfortable. You need to get as much rest as possible now; whenever you can, sit with your feet up.

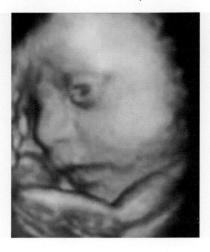

Your baby sleeps for most of the day – about 90 to 95 percent of the time, but when he's awake, he opens and closes his eyes.

BASIC LAYETTE

Although it's tempting to splurge on a wide range of cute baby clothes for your newborn, in reality your baby is likely to outgrow any first size clothes very quickly. It's best to keep these to a minimum. Buy tops with wide, envelope necks, and stretch suits or bottoms with snaps up the front and around the crotch; these are easy to put on and take off. Choose natural fibers as these minimize sweating and irritation. Suggested purchases include:

- 4 stretch suits
- 2 sleep suits
- 4 cotton undershirts
- 3 open-fronted sweaters
- 2 bibs
- 2 shawls
- Hat
- Mittens

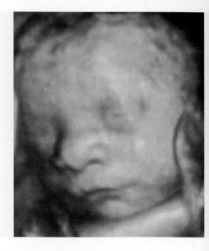

Although your baby's position has not changed in these pictures, he has probably turned head down in the uterus in preparation for birth.

DIAPERS

The first choice you'll have to make is whether you want to use disposables or washable diapers, or a combination of the two.

Disposables work by drawing moisture away from the skin into an absorbent material so that the baby's bottom remains dry. Dirty disposables are wrapped and thrown away.

Washables are made from cloth, such as toweling, and are either flat – you fold them to the required shape yourself – or pre-shaped, or come as an all-in-one system (with waterproof lining). The diapers are held in place with clips, Velcro-type fastenings or snaps. All washables, except the all-in-one system, require waterproof wraps or pants and one-way disposable liners. Dirty washables can be washed and re-used.

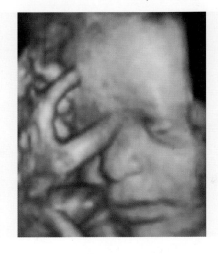

Arms, legs, and body are continuing to fill out and they are proportional to your baby's head. He makes a lot of vigorous movements now.

BABY'S ROOM

Planning and preparing the nursery is something you and your partner can share, and is one of the most enjoyable things you can do in pregnancy. When you decorate, bear in mind that your baby will quickly grow into a toddler; keep the decoration simple so that it can be changed as she grows.

Walls should be washable, so use paint rather than wallpaper and add colorful touches with peel-off stickers and stencils that can easily be updated. Invest in a blackout blind to block out the light for daytime naps, and put in a dimmer switch so you can have low-level lighting for night-time feeds.

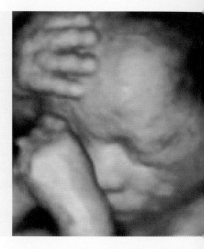

Rapid eye movements (REM) associated with dreaming can be detected now. Dreaming encourages the development of the brain, which is why your baby probably spends the majority of his time sleeping.

BABY'S CRIB

Whether you intend putting your baby in a crib straight away, or you prefer to use a Moses basket or cradle for the first few months, it's worth shopping around for one now as it may need to be ordered.

Look for a crib with a drop side so you don't strain your back bending over to pick up your baby. Some cribs also have adjustable mattress positions; the mattress can be lowered as your baby grows.

Always buy a new mattress and check that it fits snugly – the gaps around the sides should be no bigger than 1½ inches (4 cm).

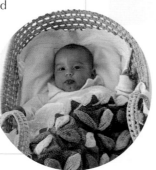

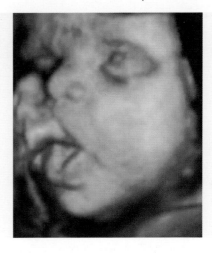

Your baby is practicing breathing movements – though he's only taking in amniotic fluid. These movements help his lungs to strengthen and develop. The fluid passes out from his bladder.

BATHING AND CHANGING EQUIPMENT

Although most newborns need only sponging down to clean them, you might like to have all your equipment on hand before baby comes home.

For bathing, most people choose portable baths, which can be placed on a firm surface at waist level. If you buy a bath stand, make sure it is very stable. Most baths come with a non-slippery surface but if yours does not, you can add a rubber mat for extra traction.

It's also important to have a special changing area set up. This could be a purpose-built unit or the top of a chest of drawers. It should have storage space for diapers and cleaning supplies.

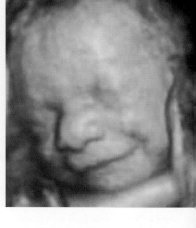

All your baby's senses are fully developed – he can hear, see, taste, smell, and touch. His sex organs are also complete; if he's a boy, both testicles should be in his scrotum.

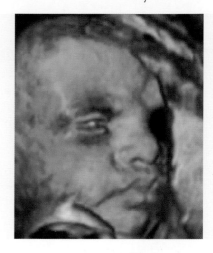

SLEEPING SAFELY

Although sudden infant death syndrome (SIDS) is thankfully rare, it's important to know what safety precautions you'll need to take to minimize any risk to your baby. It's best if your baby sleeps in your room, in a separate crib, for the first six months.

Always put her to sleep on her back, with her feet at the bottom on the crib and the covers tucked in no higher than her chest. Don't use duvets, pillows, or crib bumpers. Use a wall thermometer to keep a check on the room temperature which should be between 61 to 68°F (16 to 20°C) so she doesn't become overheated.

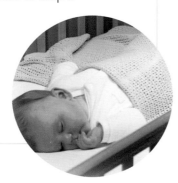

Vital Statistics

Your baby measures about 11½ inches (29 cm) from crown to rump and weighs approximately 4 pounds (1.8 kg).

33rd Week of Pregnancy

Because of her increased size, your baby's movements can be uncomfortable. You'll notice that she's very energetic and you may even feel her feet getting caught under your ribs as she twists and turns. These movements are a sign that your baby is in good health; any obvious reduction in them should be reported to your healthcare provider immediately.

As you mentally and physically prepare for the birth, sex is likely to seem less important. However, you will still need a lot of cuddles and reassurance from your partner. As long as its comfortable, it's perfectly safe to have sex throughout the last trimester unless you previously had a premature delivery, have any bleeding, or are experiencing any signs of early labor.

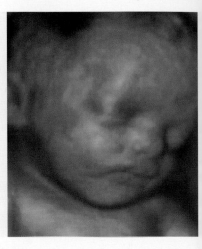

Babies in the uterus have a great many expressions. Though some scientists claim they are only reflex movements, it is difficult not to interpret them as signs of pleasure or displeasure.

CARRIAGES AND STROLLERS

Order the model you want well in advance of your due date; this is one item you won't want to be without. Think about your lifestyle – where you live and your usual way of getting around – when deciding. If you walk everywhere, a carriage with good maneuverability and suspension is a good choice. If you use the car a lot, you'll need a stroller that folds down and fits in the trunk. If you use public transport, you'll want a lightweight stroller that folds up easily and can be carried single-handedly.

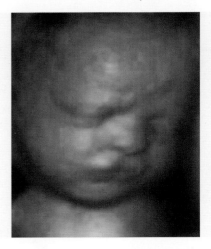

Your baby's head will increase in size by about half an inch this week due to rapid brain growth. His head is now in the correct proportion to his body.

INFANT CAR SEATS

This is an essential purchase before the birth because you'll need a car seat to bring your baby home from the hospital. The car seat must be suitable for your child's weight – weight is more important than age. Always buy new, and look for the symbol that indicates that the seat meets the current safety standard. You must get the car seat installed correctly, so find a store that offers a fitting service. Not all car seats fit all cars; check that the seat you are going to buy is suitable for your vehicle.

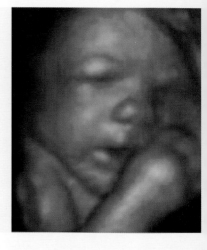

The mechanism that controls your baby's body temperature is beginning to function, and he's accumulating much more fat. However, it will be some while after birth before temperature regulation is established.

BABY PRODUCTS

Only ever use bath and cleansing products on your baby that have been specially formulated for babies. Products produced for adults may be too harsh for your baby's delicate skin.

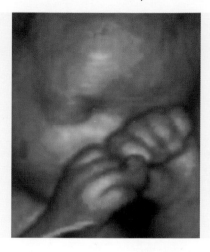

Until she reaches around three months, it's best not to use bath products or soaps when cleansing her – plain water is all that's needed at this age. Dry skin can be treated with baby oil or moisturizer, and her skin should be protected from the sun with a total UV protection cream. Avoid baby powder as some evidence suggests that inhaling it could put babies at risk.

Your baby will increasingly make more of the gestures of a full-term infant. A wide yawn is well within his capabilities.

FINANCIAL CONSIDERATIONS

By now you will either have left work, or will soon be leaving to take your maternity leave. It's a good idea to sit down and work out the financial implications that this will have on your life.

Work out the difference between the loss of income during your maternity leave and any benefits you are going to receive. If your budget is going to be tighter than you'd like, consider ways to save money, such as buying some baby items secondhand. If you're thinking about returning to work after you've had your baby, you'll need to weigh up the cost of childcare against your salary.

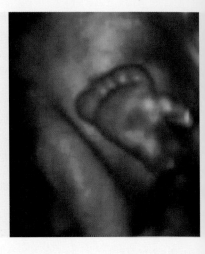

Sticking out the tongue is common fetal behavior. Your baby may be testing or tasting his environment in similar ways.

SITTING COMFORTABLY

It can be hard to get comfortable now; you are likely to be experiencing aches and pains and other discomforts of late pregnancy. Try sitting in a comfortable chair and resting your feet on a large cushion or stool. Place a cushion behind your lower back and another behind your head for support. Gradually tense and then relax all the parts of your body, starting with your head and working down to your feet. Once you are completely relaxed, breathe gently and feel yourself sinking into the comfort of the chair as you exhale.

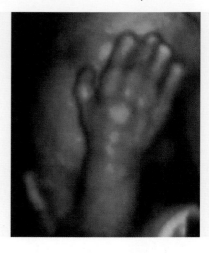

Your baby is starting to store the minerals iron, calcium, and phosphorus, which are important to his bone development.

BACKACHE

Back discomfort during pregnancy occurs when your joints are more relaxed than usual, and this along with your growing abdomen puts your body out of balance. You can try to avoid back discomfort by paying attention to your posture.

Make sure that when you sit, the chair gives your back support. Sleeping on a firm mattress with a pillow between your knees and another under your bump will give your back support at night.

Always bend from the knees when you have to lift something from the floor. If you are carrying bags, make sure that the weight is evenly distributed between your two hands. Back pain can be soothed with heat, and massage can be effective, too.

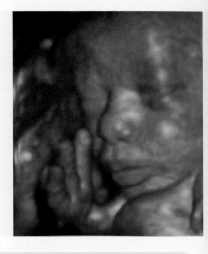

Vital Statistics

Your baby is about 12 inches (30 cm) from crown to rump and weighs approximately 4½ pounds (2 kg).

34th Week of Pregnancy

You'll be gaining around a pound a week from now until your baby is born. All the extra weight you are carrying is likely to be slowing you down, so try not to over-exert yourself and try to avoid doing unnecessary jobs.

Due to her increasing size, your baby has less room in which to move around in the uterus, but you will probably be able to distinguish her knee or foot from her elbow even though her movements are smaller.

You may also feel your baby hiccuping – a series of small rhythmic bumps in your uterus.

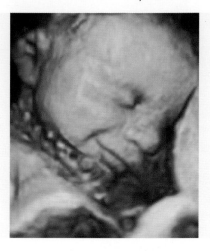

Your baby's immune system is developing rapidly; this will help him fight mild infections. It's quite common for the umbilical cord to wrap itself around your baby's neck.

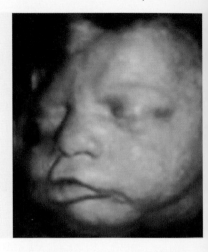

day**233**

THRUSH

Hormonal changes in pregnancy can encourage germs in the vagina to flourish, resulting in a yeast infection such as thrush. Symptoms include a thick, curd-like white discharge and a red, burning, and itchy vulva. Although thrush won't affect your pregnancy, if left untreated your baby can contract oral thrush while passing through the birth canal.

Thrush can be cured easily with vaginal creams, suppositories, or oral medicine. If you are affected by thrush, ask your healthcare provider for advice. You can help prevent thrush by eating plain yogurt with active cultures every day and cutting down on carbohydrates and sugar as these encourage yeast growth.

Your baby is capable of making a great many expressions and it can be hard not to attribute them to feelings that maturer beings exhibit. Your baby, like this one, may be getting impatient to be born.

REFLEXOLOGY

This therapy works on the principle that points on the hands and feet correspond with different parts of the body. Applying pressure to these points brings about relaxation, balance, and healing.

Reflexology can be useful in treating pregnancy symptoms such as backache, circulatory problems, and insomnia; may be employed to bring on the birth; and also can be used in labor to ease the pain of contractions.

You need to consult a qualified therapist who is experienced in the treatment of pregnant women as some pressure points, such as those that correspond with the ovaries and uterus, need to be avoided.

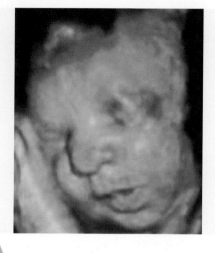

Smiling is common fetal behavior and is, surprisingly, the only form of behavior not demonstrated immediately after birth. It can take up to six weeks before your newborn smiles.

INSOMNIA

You may be feeling incredibly tired but find it hard to drop off to sleep, or find that you wake frequently during the night. Your sleep disruption may be due to physical discomforts and an inability to switch off mentally.

Try to develop a winding-down routine before bedtime. Take a candle-lit bath with a few drops of diluted lavender oil added to the water to make you feel sleepy, then lie on the sofa and listen to soothing music. Sip a milky drink before going to bed. Once in bed, make yourself comfortable by tucking a number of pillows under your bump and between your legs. Avoid watching TV too close to bedtime as it will over-stimulate your brain.

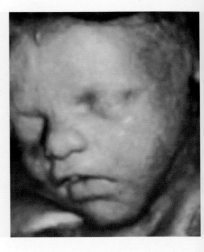

It is becoming more difficult for your baby to float in the amniotic fluid. Although he makes fewer movements, they are powerful and sustained.

NAVEL CHANGES

As your abdomen expands, you may notice that your navel changes shape. If it was concave to start with, by the middle of the pregnancy it is likely to become flat. In the last months, your growing abdomen pushes it out, so for the first time you will have an "outie." After delivery, within a few months, your navel will return to it's familiar shape.

If your navel is pierced, you may be more comfortable with the piercing removed. You shouldn't have any piercings undertaken during pregnancy because of the high risk of infection.

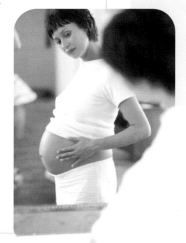

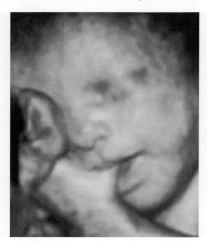

Although you can't see or feel them, your baby is capable of sustained sucking. He is honing his survival skills.

WOMB MUSIC

Your baby can hear clearly from about the 20th week of pregnancy. Research suggests that babies will remember music that they've heard in the womb up to the age of 12 months. Crying babies are often soothed by music that was played to them before they were born.

Try different types of music to see how your baby responds – she may become stimulated and excited or sedated and relaxed. Choral and piano music have patterns closest to human speech and are especially enjoyable for a baby. Your baby is receptive to your moods so play music that you enjoy so that she can pick up on this emotion from you, too.

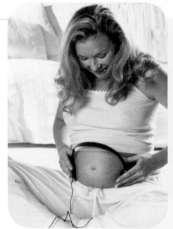

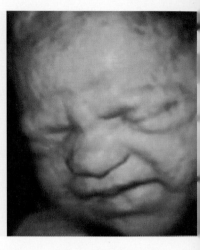

Although it has been claimed that babies cry in the uterus, this hasn't been proved scientifically. What is irrefutable, however, is that babies definitely show unhappiness and displeasure.

ABDOMINAL STRETCHING

Sometimes called hot spots, this is an uncomfortable burning sensation across your taut abdomen caused by the pressure your uterus is putting on your abdominal muscles. The pain is superficial – if you experience pain deep within your abdomen you should tell your healthcare provider immediately. Hot spots can be irritated by tight or heavy clothing, so avoid putting on pantyhose and wear loose, light garments that won't put any pressure on your abdomen. Applying an ice pack can help relieve the burning sensation.

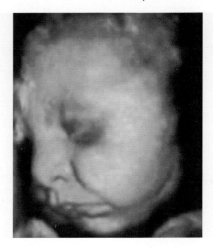

Vital Statistics

Your baby measures about 12¾ inches (32 cm) from crown to rump and weighs approximately 5 pounds (2.3 kg).

35th Week of Pregnancy

The amount of blood in your body has increased by 50 percent during the first two trimesters, but now that you've reached the 35th week, your blood volume will remain the same until you give birth.

Braxton Hicks contractions come more regularly and you may be concerned that they are the start of labor. This is rarely the case, but if the contractions are accompanied by your waters breaking then this is a cause for concern, and you will need to see your healthcare provider immediately.

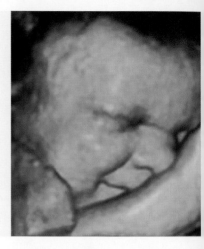

If your baby were to be born this week, he has an excellent chance of surviving without any major problems.

PERINEAL MASSAGE

This massage involves the gentle pulling down and out of the perineum – the area between the vagina and anus – to prepare it for birth. Wash your hands and then sit comfortably, with a towel under your hips. Rub a non-petroleum lubricant, such as K-Y jelly, on to your hands and the perineum and then place your thumbs 1 to 1½ inches inside your vagina. Press gently down and to the sides until you feel a slight tingling sensation. Hold the pressure for 2 minutes and then gently massage back and forth for a further 3 to 4 minutes.

Research suggests that perineal massage can help to reduce tears, the need for an episiotomy, and medical interventions such as forceps or ventouse.

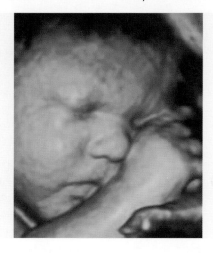

Your baby's lungs should be fully mature. Now when he breathes he produces surfactant, a protein that lowers surface tension and is essential for his lungs' healthy development.

BREECH TILT

If your baby has settled with her bottom down, practicing the breech tilt for several weeks may help her turn so that she is in the head down position. Start by getting on your hands and knees and breathing deeply for a few minutes. Then lie down with enough pillows under your pelvis to raise it to a height of 9 to 10 inches above your head. Stay in this position for 10 minutes, twice a day. Your healthcare provider will check you regularly to see if your baby has turned. If she turns, stop doing the breech tilt and start walking frequently to encourage her to remain head down.

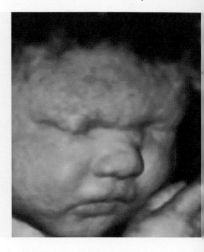

Your baby is getting plumper and plumper as he acquires more body fat. This week he will put on about half a pound but his increase in length will be minimal.

TAILOR SITTING

This exercise will release tension in your lower back and improve pelvic flexibility in preparation for the birth.

Place pillows under your thighs and sit with your back straight and the soles of your feet together. Draw your heels toward you, using your arms to push down on your thighs. Relax your shoulders and the back of your neck and breathe deeply. Hold the stretch for a count of 12. Repeat every day. As you become more flexible you will be able to remove the pillows and push your knees closer to the floor.

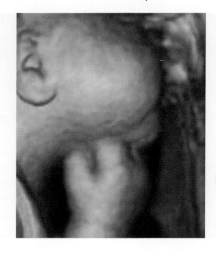

Your baby's central nervous system is maturing and he is increasingly awake and aware of his immediate environment.

PELVIC ROCKS

This is a good way to relieve backache in late pregnancy and during labor. Be careful not to let your lower back sag while doing this exercise.

Get down on your hands and knees, with your knees about hip-width apart. Keep your neck in line with your spine and your back flat. Then tighten your abdomen and buttocks and slowly round your shoulders and back and let your head drop down. Hold briefly before returning to the start position. Repeat 10 times a day or whenever you feel tension.

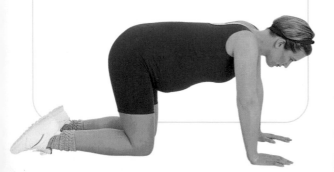

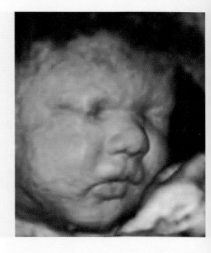

Your baby's digestive system is almost complete. He is also taking up most of the uterus and there's hardly any room for him to move about.

MODIFIED SQUATS

This exercise will strengthen your thigh muscles and encourage your baby to descend into the pelvis.

Stand with your feet hip-width apart about 2 feet from a wall. With your back and arms flat against the wall, slowly lower yourself down until your thighs are almost parallel to the floor. Make sure your knees don't go beyond your toes. Hold briefly, then slowly stand up. Repeat 12 times, twice a day.

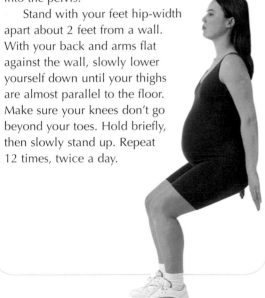

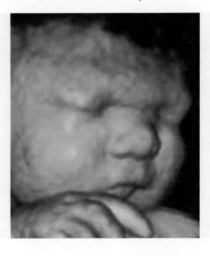

Your baby's head has probably settled near your pelvis; it is round, firm, and – if you gently push it down – it will bounce back without the rest of his body moving.

POWER KEGELS

These pelvic floor exercises will help prepare the birth canal for the delivery of your baby. You can perform them sitting, lying, or standing but not while you're urinating, as this may cause an infection,

Draw up and tighten the muscles around the anal sphincter; then hold. Slowly tighten the muscles around the urinary sphincter as well and lift up through the vagina (as though you were ascending in an elevator). Hold for a count of 6, release with control, then repeat – beginning with 4 sets of 4 reps and working up to 4 sets of 6 reps.

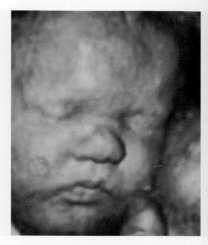

Vital Statistics

Your baby is about 13¼ inches (33 cm) from crown to rump and weighs approximately 5½ pounds (2.55 kg).

36th Week of Pregnancy

Your pelvic joints are expanding in readiness for the birth so you may be experiencing aches and pains in this area. The weight of your baby will also be putting pressure on your pelvis and the nerves in your legs, which can cause further discomfort.

You should avoid sitting or standing in one position for any length of time and should try to get plenty of rest. If you have already started your maternity leave, you may be getting bored with waiting for your baby to arrive. Try to make the most of this time by doing activities that you enjoy, such as spending time with girlfriends, or going out with your partner. Once your baby has arrived your free time will be much more limited.

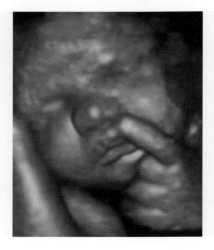

Your baby has probably reached his birth length. From now on, he'll spend his time gaining weight. He'll add around half a pound in weight in each of the subsequent weeks.

RESTLESS LEG SYNDROME

Some women develop restless leg syndrome (RLS) during pregnancy, often in the last trimester. You have an overwhelming urge to move your legs because of a crawling or tingling sensation inside your foot, calf, or upper leg, or you may feel cramping, burning, or pain in these areas. The feeling often gets worse in the evening and at night. Although not serious, this condition can be very irritating.

Stretching and rubbing your legs will bring temporary relief. Some experts believe that pregnancy-induced iron deficiency can cause, or aggravate, RLS, so discuss the problem with your healthcare provider, who may recommend an iron supplement.

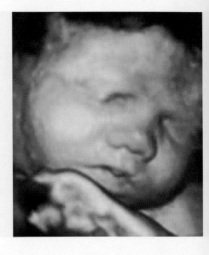

Your baby's kidneys are fully developed and his liver is able to process some waste products.

ENGAGEMENT

Toward the end of pregnancy the lower part of the uterus softens and expands allowing your baby's head to drop deeper into the pelvis. This is often referred to as the baby's head becoming "engaged" or "dropping." If you're a first-time mom this is likely to happen several weeks before the birth, although it can occur as late as the onset of labor. When this happens, some of the pressure is taken off your lungs and digestive system so your breathing becomes easier and any indigestion starts to improve.

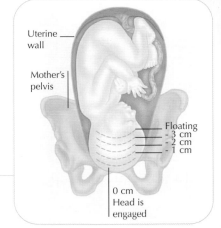

Uterine wall

Mother's pelvis

Floating
- 3 cm
- 2 cm
- 1 cm

0 cm
Head is engaged

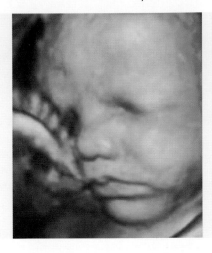

Your baby probably recognizes your voice – its qualities, tones, and rhythms – and can distinguish it from other sounds.

PROLACTIN
This is a pregnancy hormone that helps to prepare your breasts for breastfeeding. After the birth, prolactin helps to maintain your milk supply. Prolactin levels rise during the third trimester, but high levels of the hormone progesterone suppress milk production. Once progesterone levels drop after the birth, prolactin initiates the production of colostrum, your baby's first milk. Prolactin is then released in response to your baby's sucking action, enabling your breasts to produce breast milk.

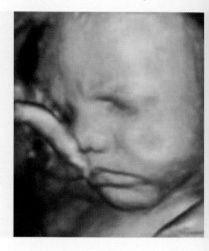

Because your baby is awake more of the time, he shows a greater range of facial expressions.

LA LECHE LEAGUE

Breastfeeding is a skill, and like any skill it has to be learned. Although your healthcare provider will be able to give you information about breastfeeding, you may find it useful to talk to other moms who have found breastfeeding a satisfying and rewarding experience.

La Leche League was set up by a group of mothers to help other moms learn to breastfeed. Its aim is to promote a better understanding of the importance of breastfeeding to the healthy development of both the baby and mother. It offers mother-to-mother support, encouragement, information, and education. La Leche League run local groups, so you may want to think about joining one in your area.

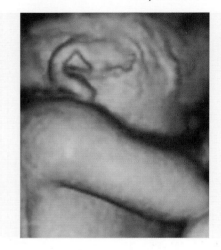

The wrinkled skin on a baby's scalp is probably due to the softness of the skull bones, which allow for further brain development and an easier passage down the birth canal. But the restricted space in the uterus may also be having an effect.

HOSPITAL BAG

Several weeks ahead of your due date, pack your bag. If you go into labor early, you'll have everything ready. How many of each you bring depends on how long you'll be in the hospital. Items you will need include:

- Robe, front-opening nightgown, and slippers
- Maternity sanitary napkins and panties
- Nursing bra and breast pads
- Toiletries and hair brush
- Cell phone and phone numbers for after the birth
- Money
- Camera and video equipment
- Watch with a second hand for timing contractions
- Socks for cold feet

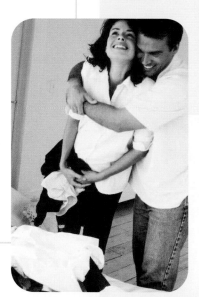

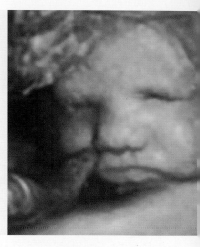

Your baby's lungs should be mature enough so that he can breathe unaided if born now. Maturity depends on having sufficient surfactant, a protein that enables his lungs to expand.

BREATHING TECHNIQUES

At prenatal classes you will be shown breathing techniques for labor and birth. Learning how to breathe deeply in a controlled, calm way will help your muscles relax, slow down your heart rate, and give you something on which to focus. Shallow, panicky breathing can restrict the oxygen supply to your muscles and increase cramping and pain, and may even make you lightheaded.

Spend time practicing your breathing techniques with your birth partner so that he or she can help you with them if you forget what you are supposed to be doing during the birth.

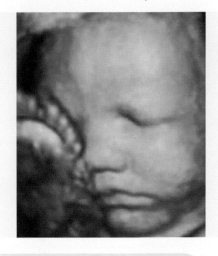

Vital Statistics

Your baby measures about 13½ inches (34 cm) from crown to rump and weighs approximately 6 pounds (2.75 kg).

37th Week of Pregnancy

You'll be attending prenatal checks every week now and your healthcare provider will feel your abdomen to check your baby's position at each visit. Your uterus has reached it highest point, just below your breastbone, and your breasts are getting bigger and heavier.

Make sure your hospital bag is packed and think about any labor aids you may want to take with you, such as a birthing ball or extra pillows. If you are planning to use alternative therapies during labor, talk to your therapist about anything special you may need to have on hand.

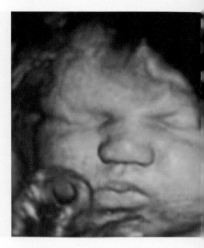

From now on, your baby can be born at almost any time. No one, however, knows what triggers labor. Some scientists believe it is secretions from your baby's adrenal glands that initiate the process.

PRENATAL "BLUES"

It's quite normal to feel anxious and a bit "down" at times during pregnancy, and these feelings are especially common during the last six weeks. You'll be physically exhausted, as well as naturally concerned about the birth and how you will cope with labor. Any depression is usually short-lived and may be helped by getting more rest. Keep activities to a minimum, and try to have a nap during the middle of the day and get to bed early. Don't bottle-up how you are feeling – talk to your partner, mom, or healthcare provider. They will be able to reassure you.

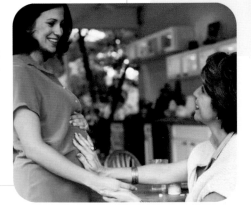

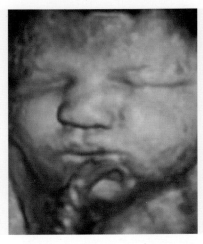

Your baby's immune system continues to develop in order to protect him once he's born. Antibodies he doesn't produce himself he'll receive from you via the placenta.

KICK CHART

As birth approaches, it's a good idea to keep track of your baby's movements as activity levels are good indicators of her well-being.

Fill out a kick chart each day to record any wriggling, punching or kicking over a number of hours. If you notice any significant reduction in movement – whether or not you've been filling in a kick chart – you should tell your healthcare provider immediately.

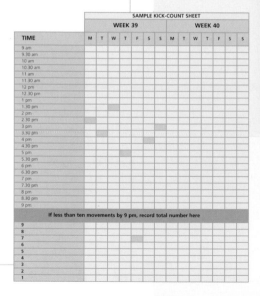

SAMPLE KICK-COUNT SHEET													
	WEEK 39						WEEK 40						
TIME	M	T	W	T	F	S	S	M	T	W	T	F	S	S
9 am														
9.30 am														
10 am														
10.30 am														
11 am														
11.30 am														
12 pm														
12.30 pm														
1 pm														
1.30 pm														
2 pm														
2.30 pm														
3 pm														
3.30 pm														
4 pm														
4.30 pm														
5 pm														
5.30 pm														
6 pm														
6.30 pm														
7 pm														
7.30 pm														
8 pm														
8.30 pm														
9 pm														
If less than ten movements by 9 pm, record total number here														
9														
8														
7														
6														
5														
4														
3														
2														
1														

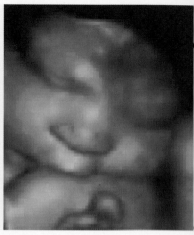

Sucking is fully established and your baby will latch on to any body part that comes close.

GETTING TO THE HOSPITAL

You'll need to sort out your travel arrangements for getting to the hospital well before your due date. If you are going by car, it's worth trying the journey at different times of the day to see what the traffic is like.

Find out about parking; your partner will probably have to leave the car for longer than a few hours, so you'll need to check out the time limits and parking charges of local lots.

If you plan to use a taxi firm, make sure it is reliable and have the phone number of a second taxi company as backup.

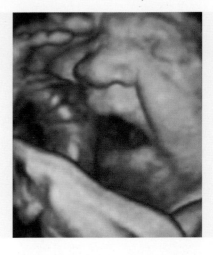

Your baby now spends about 30 percent of the time in quiet sleep and 60 percent in active sleep, when eye and body movements occur, and the heart rate speeds up. 10 percent of the time he is awake, with eyes and limbs moving continually.

NESTING INSTINCT

This is a sudden burst of energy, which often occurs in the weeks before the birth, and may become stronger a few days before labor starts. You may find that you have a sudden urge to start clearing out cupboards, washing curtains, and generally doing jobs you haven't had the energy for in the last few months.

The nesting instinct is often seen as an in-built maternal desire to prepare the home for the imminent arrival of the baby. Make the most of this burst of energy, but don't tire yourself out – you'll need all your strength for labor.

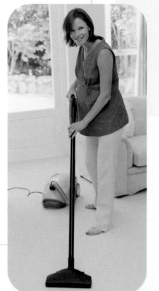

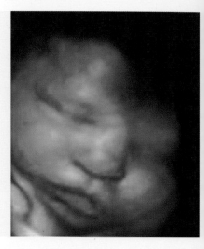

Almost all the lanugo hair has disappeared from your baby's body, but he has head hair, which varies from a few strands on the back of his head to a thick mop about an inch long.

STAGES OF CHILDBIRTH

There are three stages of childbirth. The first and longest stage is labor, when uterine contractions dilate the cervix so that your baby can pass out of the uterus into the birth canal.

The second stage, which can take from 10 minutes up to three hours, is the birth of your baby. During this stage, your baby is pushed down the birth canal and out through the vagina.

The third stage is the delivery of the placenta. This when the placenta detaches itself from the uterine wall and is expelled from your body. The delivery of the placenta is the easiest stage and happens relatively automatically.

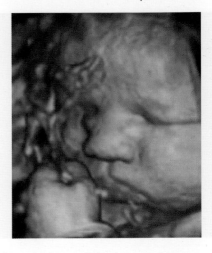

Instead of large kicks and thrusts, your baby's movements are reduced to squirming and trying to stretch out his arms and legs.

LABOR SIGNS

It's quite natural to be worried that you won't recognize when you are in labor. But the truth is that most women know as soon as labor starts. There are some classic signs to look out for that indicate that labor has begun – or is about to begin.

You may have a "show" (the expulsion of the mucus plug from the cervix), your waters may break, or you may start to experience contractions that are more regular and stronger than the Braxton Hicks contractions you've been having. These signs can happen in any order, and although they don't necessarily mean that your baby is about to be born, they are good indications that your body is getting ready for the birth.

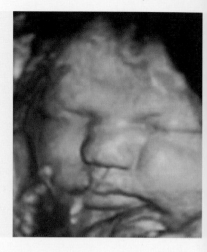

Vital Statistics
Your baby measures about 14 inches (35 cm) from crown to rump and weighs approximately 6½ pounds (2.95 kg).

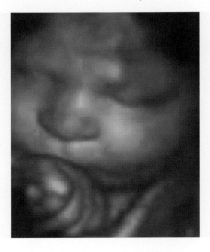

38th Week of Pregnancy

You may be feeling less pressure on your chest and stomach if your baby has moved down into the pelvis, but walking may be more uncomfortable if her head is pressing on your pelvic floor.

The uterus is putting a lot of pressure on your bladder now, so you will be making frequent trips to the bathroom.

You may be feeling more irritable than usual, because you're finding everything an effort, and this, coupled with lack of sleep and fears about the birth, can affect your mood. Tell your partner how you are feeling so that he can give you extra support during these last weeks.

Readying himself for birth, your baby engages in a lot of the activity you will see once he's born. He probably spends a lot of his awake time sucking.

POSITIONS FOR LABOR

Unless you have to be in bed for some medical reason, being active during labor will allow gravity to help your baby out. Walking or standing can be helpful during the early stages, while squatting and kneeling may be more comfortable as you near the birth.
Squat down using your birth partner for support. This position helps to widen the pelvis and encourages your baby to descend more rapidly.

If your baby is coming too fast, slow down her descent by going down on your knees and resting your arms on pillows or a bean bag.

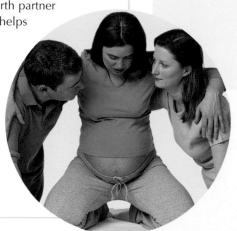

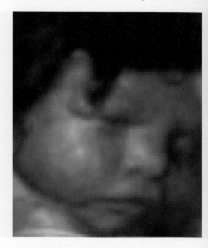

Your baby is awake more of the time. He has established his own routines of wakefulness and sleep over a 24-hour period.

BIRTH POSITIONS

You may want to try a number of different positions before you get to the pushing stage to see which is the most comfortable. Lay back with your back supported by pillows and your legs apart. This is a good position if you're tiring, or if your baby requires continuous electronic monitoring.

Lie on your side with pillows or a bean bag for support and hold your upper leg – or get your birth partner to hold it for you. This position is good if you've had an epidural, or you're tiring, because it can make the contractions more effective.

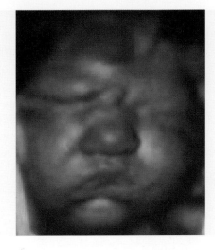

Your baby is so big that he won't be able to turn around and change his position before birth. He spends his time putting on weight.

AIDS FOR LABOR

A birthing ball, bean bag and large, comfortable pillows will help make labor more comfortable. Find out what's available to use and take anything else you need into the hospital with you. Labor rooms can be cold and unhomely so you may want a few familiar items with you for comfort and reassurance. Things you could take include:

- Calming music
- Electric aromatherapy burner with oils
- Water spray to freshen you
- Natural sponge for cooling you down
- Magazine or book
- Massage lotion
- Hot water bottle
- Snacks for you and your partner
- Flask for ice cubes
- Mirror to see baby emerge

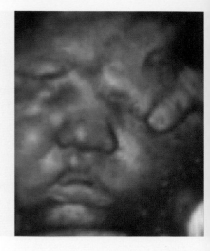

A significant proportion of your baby's expressions and movements are reactions to sound, touch, and other sensations.

DILATION & EFFACEMENT

These are words that you will hear a lot during labor. They refer to the thinning out (effacement) and opening up (dilation) of the cervix so that your baby can be born. Your cervix has been tightly closed and protected by a plug of mucus throughout your pregnancy. As labor nears, your baby's head drops down into the pelvis and pushes against the cervix, causing it to relax and thin out. After the cervix begins to efface, it also starts to open or dilate. When labor begins it may have already dilated to between 2 and 4 cm. During the course of labor it continues to dilate until it is fully open at 10 cm (4 inches).

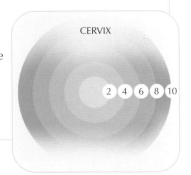

CERVIX

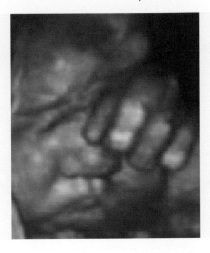

Your baby's environment is changing and we don't know how he feels about it. Early uterine contractions will be compressing the womb around him.

PRESENTATION

When contractions begin, how your baby "presents" can affect your labor. The most usual presentation is occipito anterior. This is when the baby is head down and curled into a neat little ball.

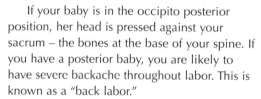

If your baby is in the occipito posterior position, her head is pressed against your sacrum – the bones at the base of your spine. If you have a posterior baby, you are likely to have severe backache throughout labor. This is known as a "back labor."

A baby in the breech position – bottom or legs down – may need to be delivered by cesarean, although vaginal birth of a breech baby is sometimes possible under the supervision of an obstetrician.

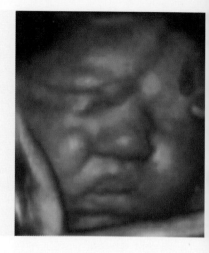

Your baby's head and abdomen have about the same circumference. Your birth practitioner could hazard a guess about how large your baby will be, but you might be in for a surprise.

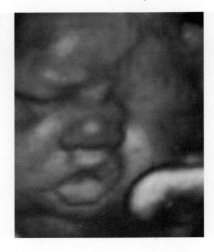

GOING HOME BAG

It's a good idea to have a bag packed with all the items you'll need for your return home. After all the excitement of the birth your partner may not be the best person to be relied on to choose the right clothes for you to wear when you leave the hospital. It's worth remembering, too, that although you will look and feel a lot slimmer, you'll still be a lot larger than your pre-pregnancy size, so pack a loose-fitting outfit and comfortable shoes. Other things to include are:

- Bag for carrying home gifts and hospital supplies
- Clothes for your baby: undershirt, stretchsuit, receiving blanket and a jacket, hat, and mittens if the weather is cold
- Diapers and baby wipes
- Infant car seat

Vital Statistics

Your baby measures 14½ inches (37 cm) from crown to rump and weighs about 6 pounds 13 ounces (3.05 kg).

39th Week of Pregnancy

You could go into labor at any time from this week on so you may be worried that you won't recognize when labor starts. This is a common fear, but it is unlikely that you won't know.

You may start to experience false labor contractions now. These are stronger than Braxton Hicks contractions, but not quite as strong as the real thing. They are not regular and usually disappear when you move about. These early contractions are preparing your uterus and softening the cervix for when labor really begins.

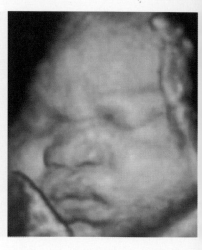

Your baby is clinically mature and can be born at any time. The placenta, which has sustained him up to now, is beginning to age and become less efficient at transferring nutrients.

PAIN RELIEF

Your choice of pain relief can make a big difference to your birth experience. If you are considering pain-relief drugs, make sure you understand what drugs are available and how they work so that when the time comes you can make an informed decision about which type of drug to have. Alternative forms of pain relief include relaxation and breathing techniques, hypnosis, acupuncture, reflexology, aromatherapy, and the use of transcutaneous electronic nerve stimulation (TENS). All of these need to be organized before the birth and in some cases you may need to have a qualified therapist with you during labor.

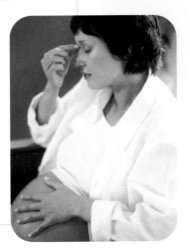

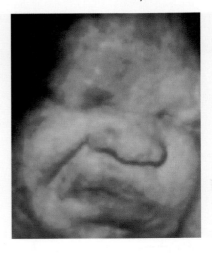

More of your antibodies cross the placental barrier and enter your baby's bloodstream in order to give his immune system a temporary boost.

TENS

Transcutaneous Electrical Nerve Stimulation
(TENS) uses a weak electrical current to block
pain messages to the brain and stimulate the
body to produce endorphins – its own natural
painkillers. A small hand-held device is
attached by four electrodes to your back. You
control the strength of the
current yourself by
turning a dial on the
machine. TENS is most
effective during early
labor and can help to
reduce backache in back
labor. Your healthcare
provider will be able to
advise you about hiring
a TENS machine for use
at home.

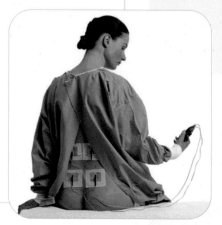

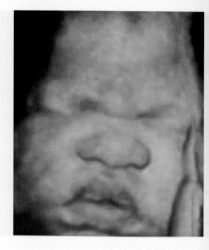

Less amniotic fluid surrounds your baby,
and the umbilical cord, which is about the
same length as your baby, will soon finish
its work.

EPIDURAL

This is a popular choice of pain relief because it is very effective. it allows you to remain awake and alert and it doesn't affect your baby. An epidural involves injecting an anesthetic into the epidural space in the lower back. It works by numbing the lower half of the body, blocking the nerves that relay pain messages back to the brain. An epidural needs to be set up by an anesthetist, which takes about 15 minutes. You will start to feel the effects within 10 to 20 minutes, and these will last for between 2 and 4 hours and can be increased if required.

Spinal cord

Epidural space

Vertebra

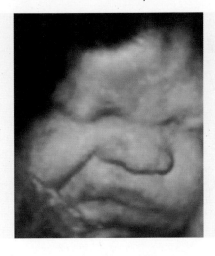

Meconium, a greenish-black sticky substance made up of waste material, is accumulating in your baby's intestines.

ANALGESICS IN LABOR

These drugs are used to help reduce the pain of contractions, but because they pass through your bloodstream, they affect your baby. The drugs are given intravenously and take effect in 2 to 15 minutes and last for 2 to 4 hours. Analgesics will relax you and take the edge off the pain, but they may make you feel sleepy and disorientated, and can make your baby drowsy. Entonox – gas and oxygen – offers more controllable short-term pain relief. It is breathed in from a machine, which you control yourself, and takes effect within 15 to 30 seconds but only lasts for up to a minute. Although Entonox passes to your baby, it is cleared from the baby's system with the first breaths she takes after the birth.

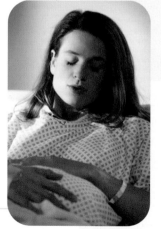

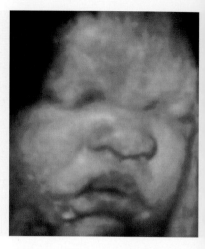

Your baby's abdominal circumference is now slightly larger than his head and about 15 percent of his body is fat. All his body systems are developed.

WATER

Immersing yourself in warm water can be a surprisingly effective form of pain relief, especially when used during the last stages of labor when contractions are at their strongest. Being in water relaxes you, making contractions easier to bear. It also supports you, so that moving into different positions becomes easier. Some studies report that water reduces blood pressure, speeds up the dilation of the cervix, and helps the baby to descend more rapidly. The use of water often reduces the need for other forms of pain relief.

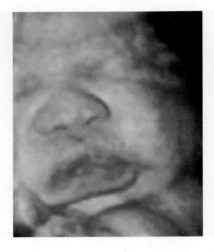

Gravity and the fact that your baby is now probably quite far down in your pelvic girdle means that his head is being compressed to a certain degree.

YOUR PARTNER AND LABOR

Giving emotional support, massage, and help with breathing and relaxation techniques are just some of the ways your birth partner can support you through the birth. It's important that your partner has a clear understanding before labor begins as to how you'd like it to be managed. Go through your birth plan together and talk through any concerns or fears you may have. This will make it easier for your partner to interpret your wishes so that he or she can give you the best possible assistance when you most need it.

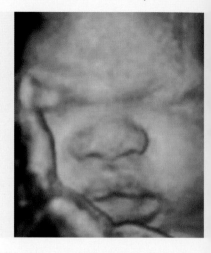

Vital Statistics
Your baby measures about 21½ inches (48 cm) in total and weighs approximately 7 pounds (3.25 kg).

FINAL WEEK OF PREGNANCY?

You've now reached the 40th week of pregnancy and the likely time of your baby's birth, though only around 5 percent of babies are born exactly on their EDD.

Your weight is likely to plateau now, and you may even lose a few pounds. Your uterus is taking up all the space in your pelvis and a lot of room in your abdomen, so you will be feeling extremely uncomfortable.

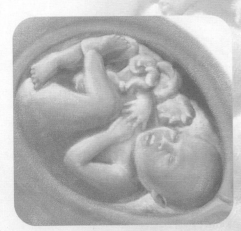

As you near your due date you may want to try making love to encourage labor to start. Having sex releases the hormone oxytocin into your bloodstream, which ripens the cervix. Orgasm may also help to start contractions. Any lovemaking needs to be very gentle as it could be very uncomfortable for both you and your baby.

A "SHOW"

Your cervix has been sealed with a mucus plug throughout your pregnancy. As the cervix begins to stretch and soften, this plug is dislodged and appears from the vagina as a bloodstained mucus discharge. This is known as a "show." Although a show is often a sign that labor is imminent, it can also appear two to three weeks before labor begins, or it may not come out until contractions are well underway so that you don't even notice it. Tell your healthcare provider when you have a show so that you can be assessed to see whether labor is starting.

RUPTURE OF MEMBRANES

The membranes that hold the amniotic fluid that protects your baby in the uterus usually break early in labor. This is known as the "waters breaking." If this happens before labor starts – premature rupture of the membranes – you are likely to go into labor within the next 24 hours. You will experience your waters breaking as either a trickle or a gush of clear, odorless fluid from the vagina. If the liquid is yellow, greenish, or brown you should contact your healthcare provider immediately, as this may mean your baby is in distress. If your waters break at home you need to inform your healthcare provider.

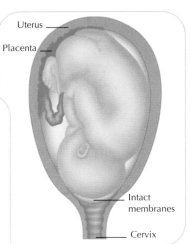

Uterus

Placenta

Intact membranes

Cervix

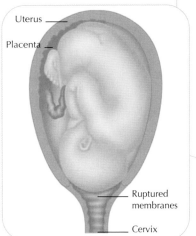

Uterus

Placenta

Ruptured membranes

Cervix

CONTRACTIONS

When you are in true labor your contractions become symmetrical – starting at the cervix, moving up and around to the back, or from the back to the front. They are regular and in a predictable pattern and as labor progresses they get longer and stronger and closer together. During the early stage, contractions last for 30 to 45 seconds and can range from 20 to five minutes apart. As labor advances their intensity picks up and they start coming every two to three minutes, and last for 30 seconds to one minute. You need to time your contractions, and when they are coming regularly, at five minute intervals, you will need to go to the hospital. True labor begins when the contractions become regular and longer lasting. These more powerful contractions squeeze your baby down on to the cervix so that the pressure from her head gradually effaces (thins) and dilates (opens) it. By the end of the first stage of childbirth the cervix will have dilated to 4 inches (10 cms).

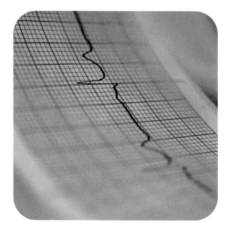

FETAL MONITORING

Your healthcare provider will want to monitor your baby's progress during labor. Some hospitals carry out continuous monitoring, others use fetal monitoring intermittently. This can be done with an external fetal monitor which gives readings of your baby's heartbeat and your contractions. Some healthcare providers measure a baby's progress with a hand-held ultrasound device called a doppler. If there is reason for concern, internal monitoring – an electrode is attached to your baby's scalp – may be used. Although this is a more accurate type of monitoring, it does restrict your mobility and there is a slight risk of your baby getting an infection from the electrode.

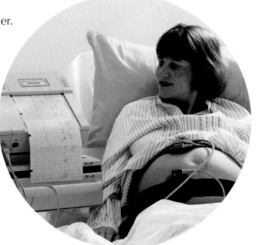

BIRTH

You may feel a renewed burst of energy once you know the end of labor is in sight, and you will have an overwhelming urge to push. Each contraction pushes your baby a little bit further down the vagina until her head arrives at the vaginal opening – this is known as "crowning." You'll feel an intense burning and pressure on your rectum as your baby's head pushes against the perineum. Your healthcare provider will ask you to pant rather than push so that the perineum can stretch as your baby's head is delivered. The next contractions will deliver the shoulders and then the rest of your baby's body will immediately follow.

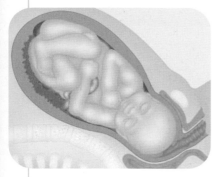 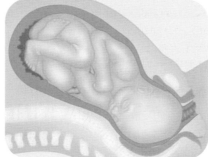 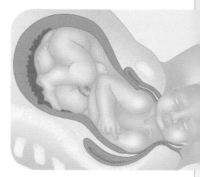

THE FINAL STAGES

Once he's born, your baby will be given an identity anklet and bracelet, and his umbilical cord will be clamped and cut. After a brief check, your baby will be handed to you. Lay him on his stomach so he can be comforted by your heartbeat and breathing rhythmns, which will be familiar to him.

Delivery of the placenta

After the delivery of your baby, further contractions separate your placenta from the uterine wall. You may be offered an injection of syntocinon or syntometrine, drugs that speed up the delivery of the placenta and reduce postpartum bleeding. If you want the delivery to be natural, your healthcare provider may massage your uterus and gently pull on the umbilical cord as you push the placenta out. Once delivered, the placenta will be checked to make sure it is whole and that nothing has been left in the uterus. It's quite normal to experience some severe shaking and shivering after your placenta is delivered.

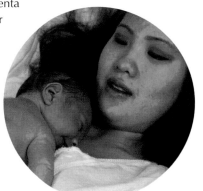

HOME BIRTH

If you are having your baby at home, your midwife will normally be with you throughout your labor but will not interfere unless he or she suspects complications. There will be no intervention of any type and you will be encouraged to deal with the pain of contractions through breathing, possibly the use of water, adopting different positions – almost anything that makes you feel more comfortable. The midwife will provide encouragement and information about the baby's progress down the birth canal, and can answer any questions you may have about the procedure.

Most midwives feel their role is to let the mother deliver her baby; they are there to receive the baby and ensure that should help be needed, they can provide the backup or transport the mother to the hospital.

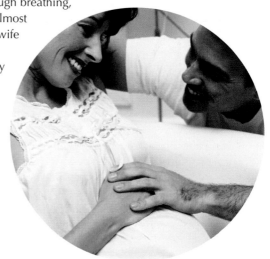

CESAREAN DELIVERY

You will be offered a regional (epidural or spinal block) or general anesthetic depending upon your condition. If you have a regional anesthetic, you will be awake. The area of your abdomen where the incision will be made will be preped, and you will have a bladder catheter inserted to drain urine.

Generally, the abdominal area will be screened from your view. The surgeon will make an incision through your lower abdomen, and will push aside the muscles there and possibly the bladder. Then another incision will be made in the uterus. As the amniotic fluid is drained, you may hear a whooshing noise. You may then feel some pressure and a tugging sensation as your baby is lifted out through the incision.

The surgeon will then remove the placenta and will sew closed your uterus and the layers of your abdominal wall. Your skin will be closed with either dissolvable sutures or staples.

You will be handed your baby and, once both of you are ready to be moved, you will be taken to a recovery unit.

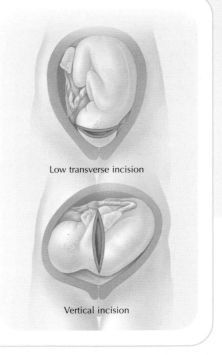

Low transverse incision

Vertical incision

FORCEPS DELIVERY

If for any reason you can't push the baby out, or your baby needs to be born quickly, forceps may be used to help deliver her. Forceps are medical instruments that look like a large pair of salad servers. After an episiotomy, the forceps are inserted into the vagina and are cupped around the baby's head. During a contraction, you will push while your healthcare provider gently pulls the baby down the birth canal. Once the head is born, you should be able to deliver the rest of your baby yourself. The forceps may leave marks on the sides of your baby's head, but these will soon disappear.

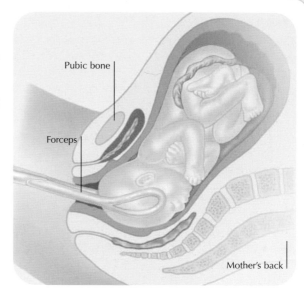

Pubic bone

Forceps

Mother's back

VENTOUSE DELIVERY

This is a type of vacuum extraction, which is used to gently suck the baby out of the birth canal. It is often used instead of forceps if there is a problem delivering the baby. It is less painful for mothers during and after birth than forceps and there is less risk of bladder or bowel damage. An episiotomy is not always required.

A soft vacuum cup is attached to the baby's head and then suction, produced by a pump, is used to pull the baby while you push during a contraction. The cup can be applied higher up the vagina than forceps so it can be attached to the baby before he starts to descend down the birth canal.

Some babies have slightly cone-shaped heads and/or a blood blister for a few days afterward.

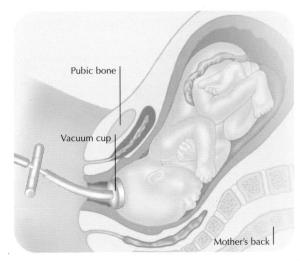

Pubic bone

Vacuum cup

Mother's back

EPISIOTOMY

This is a surgical cut that is made to enlarge the vaginal opening. It is done with scissors, under local anesthetic when the head is crowning, just before the birth. You may need an episiotomy to prevent the perineum from tearing if it hasn't stretched sufficiently to allow your baby's head to be born. If forceps or ventouse are used an episiotomy will be given. After the birth, the cut is stitched and the perineum will be sore and swollen for days, and even weeks after the birth. Your healthcare provider may give you a local anesthetic spray to apply to the area.

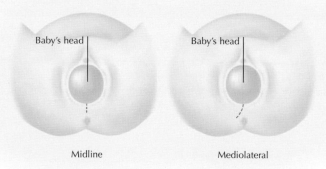

Midline   Mediolateral

MULTIPLE BIRTH

If you are expecting more than one baby, you will be advised well before your due date as to whether you can give birth naturally or if a cesarean will be required. Even if you are hoping to have a vaginal birth, a multiple birth has to take place in hospital so that a cesarean can be carried out if an emergency occurs. Twins can be delivered vaginally, often without any problems – in fact the birth tends to be faster than if you are having a single baby. If you are expecting triplets or more, then a planned cesarean is probably your only option.

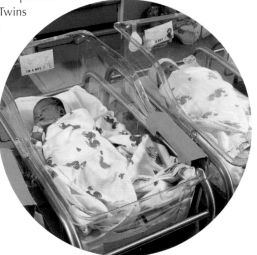

APGAR SCORE

Immediately afer the birth, your healthcare provider will carry out a quick assessment of your baby's health, known as the Apgar score. The test, devised by Dr. Virginia Apgar, is concerned with five signs. For each of these, your baby will be given a score of 0, 1, or 2. A baby rarely receives a total score of 10, but a score of 7 is generally regarded as fine. If he scores lower, he'll need some temporary medical help and close monitoring. The Apgar score is not an indicator of future health.

SIGN	POINTS		
	0	1	2
Appearance	Pale or blue	Body pink, extremities blue	Pink
Pulse	Not detectable	Below 100	Over 100
Grimace (reflexes)	No response to stimulation	Grimace	Lusty cry, cough, or sneeze
Activity (muscle tone)	Flaccid (no or weak activity)	Some movement of extremities	A lot of activity
Respiration	None	Slow, irregular	Good, crying

GOING OVERDUE

Although pregnancy is described as 40 weeks in length, only 5 percent of babies actually arrive on time, most arrive slightly late. It's perfectly normal for a baby to be born two weeks either side of the due date.

Being one or two weeks overdue is not considered a cause for concern by your healthcare providers, providing that you and your baby are well. Your healthcare provider may perform some tests, including an ultrasound to check on your baby.

Once your pregnancy reaches 42 weeks you are considered to be officially late, and you may be given a date to go into the hospital. Your healthcare provider will discuss induction with you as you approach the 42nd week, because the longer the pregnancy goes on, the less efficient the placenta becomes, so your baby could be at risk. Make sure you find out what method will be used to induce labor and how your labor is likely to progress afterward.

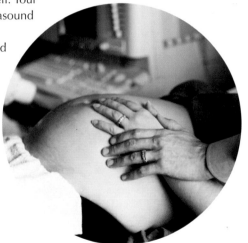

MONITORING YOUR OVERDUE BABY

Once you have passed your due date your healthcare provider will want to monitor your baby to ensure that she is still thriving. A fetal monitor will be used to check your baby's heartbeats. Your doctor may stimulate contractions and use a fetal monitor to record your baby's response to the stress of the contractions. An ultrasound may be used to measure your baby's limbs and lung movements, and the amount of amniotic fluid left in the uterus. You may also be asked to keep a kick chart to monitor her movements. If any of these tests indicate that your baby could be at risk, induction will be recommended.

If you want to avoid being artificially induced there are a number of natural things you can try to encourage labor to start. Have intercourse – semen is rich in prostaglandins, hormones that soften the cervix, while orgasm is also known to stimulate contractions. Nipple stimulation causes the secretion of oxytocin, the hormone that stimulates contractions, and these contractions will help to soften the cervix in preparation for labor.

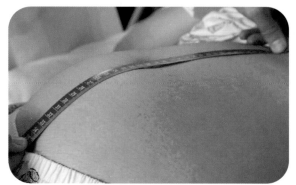

INDUCTION

Sometimes labor has to be started artificially, a procedure known as induction. This may be because you or your baby are considered at risk, or because you are overdue. Induction may be done by inserting a suppository or gel into the vagina to soften the cervix and encourage contractions to start.

Artificial rupture of the membranes (ARM) may also be carried out – the bag of membranes is punctured so that the amniotic fluid is released. Another way of inducing labor is to give a synthetic form of oxytocin, the natural hormone in your body which causes the uterus to contract (see left). Induction is planned in advance so you'll have time to discuss the method being used with your healthcare provider.

PLACENTAL ABRUPTION

Normally the placenta separates from the uterus and is delivered after the birth. Very occasionally the placenta starts to tear away from the uterus before the baby is born. Known as placental abruption, this can cause serious problems for both the mother and the baby.

Symptoms include contractions that don't stop, abdominal pain, and sometimes vaginal bleeding.

Treatment will depend on how much of the placenta has separated from the uterus, how close your pregnancy is to full term, your general health, and the health of your baby. If the separation is small and your baby isn't distressed, you may be able to continue with the pregnancy with frequent check ups. Moderate to severe placental abruption requires the immediate delivery of the baby.

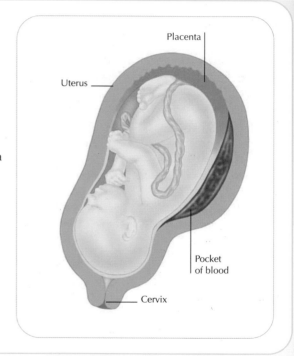

Placenta

Uterus

Pocket of blood

Cervix

PLACENTA PREVIA

You may be told that you have a low-lying placenta at your anomaly scan, but usually, during the last weeks of pregnancy, the placenta moves up and out of the way. If the placenta remains below the baby it will partially or completely block the cervix – a condition known as placenta previa.

Bleeding or spotting is usually the only symptom. Treatment will depend on the amount of blood loss and whether the cervix is partially or completely blocked. Sometimes bed rest is all that is needed, but in around 50 percent of cases, the baby has to be delivered early.

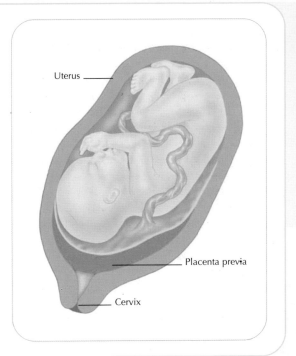

Uterus

Placenta previa

Cervix

EMERGENCY CESAREAN

This operation is carried out when a complication occurs during labor. Reasons for an emergency cesarean include problems with the placenta, such as placental abruption or placenta previa, or the baby being premature, becoming distressed, or being too big to pass through the pelvis. Sometimes, when the labor has been very long, the mother and baby become too exhausted to proceed with a vaginal delivery.

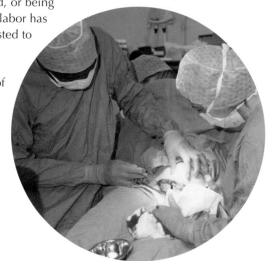

The procedure is identical to a planned cesarean but can be more stressful due to the circumstances. Instead of an epidural, you may be given a general anesthetic and the incision may be larger if the baby is in an awkward position. Your partner may be excluded from the delivery room. Your stay in hospital will be longer than if you have a vaginal delivery.

SPECIAL CARE BABIES

Babies who are too small at birth (weighing less than 5½ pounds) or who are born too early (before 37 weeks), will need to be cared for in a special care baby unit.

If your baby's lungs are still immature, he will have to be put on a ventilator and be given intravenous fluids and antibiotics to prevent infections. These will either be administered through an IV or umbilical central line.

He will be placed on a special bed with a radiant warmer to help maintain his body temperature, and a cellophane wrapping may be used to minimize the loss of heat and fluids through his skin. He may also have a feeding tube inserted and a cardiorespiratory monitor with a pulse oximeter attached to measure the oxygen in his blood.

Even if he's in an incubator, you should be able to stroke him, and many mothers express breast milk that can be used for feeding.

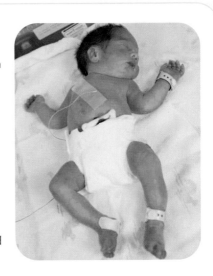

ACKNOWLEDGMENTS

PICTURE CREDITS
Illustrations by Amanda Williams

Front jacket Getty Images; p 71 (left) Simon Fraser/SPL; p 74 (left) Caroline Mardon; p 81 (left) Samuel Ashfield/SPL; p 84 (left) Mother & Baby Picture Library/Ian Hooton; p 85 (left) BSIP Vem/SPL; p 98 (left) Caroline Mardon; p 101 (left) Caroline Mardon; p 203 (left) www.thinkvegetables.co.uk:MW Mack; p 210 (left) Mother & Baby Picture Library/Ruth Jenkinson; p 242 (left) Retna/Luci Pashley; p 283 Midirs Photo Library; p 298 (left) Mother & Baby Picture Library/Frances Tout